Living Long,

Living Passionately

Also by Karen Casey

Living Long, Living Passionately

75 (and Counting) Ways to Bring Peace and Purpose to Your Life

Karen Casey

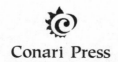

Conari Press

This edition first published in 2015 by Conari Press, an imprint of
Red Wheel/Weiser, LLC
With offices at:
665 Third Street, Suite 400
San Francisco, CA 94107
www.redwheelweiser.com

ISBN: 978-1-57324-654-5

Library of Congress Cataloging-in-Publication Data available upon request.

Cover design by Jim Warner
Cover rose photograph © Kristo Gothard Hunor / Shutterstock
Cover runner photograph © Halfpoint / Shutterstock
Interior by Jane Hagaman
Typeset in Minion Pro

Printed in the United States of America
M&G
10 9 8 7 6 5 4 3 2 1

Contents

Author's Note

Use this book as your guide and inspiration. Have a notebook or journal dedicated to the exercises you choose to do from this book. Take the book at your own pace—spend as much or as little time as you want to spend with any one topic. You can either go through from start to finish or skip around as topics appeal to your needs and interests.

Explore fear and love, resistance and acceptance, willpower and discernment. Bring peace into your daily life. This is a book to return to again and again. Savor each of the seventy-five essays and the practices that follow it. Choose the ones that speak to you and discard the rest.

Introduction

Breathe, Pause, Breathe, Pause, Breathe . . .

The gift of a somewhat retired life is having the time to fully appreciate the power of now, the power of nothingness. Which is, of course, the power of everythingness. This is a space I'm growing into in these days and weeks, hopefully months and years too, since turning seventy-five. Everythingness—what a glorious doorway to the unfolding of a life already well lived, and yet one that is ripe for far more living.

Since the age of thirteen, I have been employed. I have also been an alcoholic since that age. Until now, I had not considered that parallel in my life. Does the alcoholism in fact "complement" the work life? I think it did for me. The drink was quite often the reward for work well done. As I aged, the alcohol also fueled the act of working. Seldom did I grade papers, develop strategic plans, or study for exams without a glass of Jack Daniel's by my side. It eased the transition between thoughts and words on the page. It eased all the years it took to become a PhD.

Throughout the journey from drink number one to the celebration of thirty-eight years of abstinence, I passed through many portals of life, and seldom did I take the time to breathe, pause, and breathe again. I simply rushed by the events, the people, the inclinations to make choice A rather than choice B. I had never considered the idea that what caught my attention had been "sent" from on high.

Today, my faith is a thread that I have busily knit into the tapestry that is mine, and only mine. Knitting and breathing and pausing I know to be my main "assignments." I say assignment because that word implies a necessary act. The act of breathing is, of course, mandatory for us all. The gift of pausing is an act to be cultivated, daily, hourly, even minute by minute. Cultivated not unlike the garden of vegetables we hover over after planting, pulling the hungry weeds stealing the moisture away from the roots feeding the carrots and the lettuce and the ruby red tomatoes. And knitting? Well, knitting the myriad threads is done automatically. By you, by me, by every creature of the forests and the streams.

The many flowers along the side of one's house scream for our attention in the midst of the breathing and pausing that have become our work, as the years draw us into the future moments, moments that have our names indelibly etched on them. Having these future moments call me to attention is one of the rewards of a life well lived, a life that has learned to be willing to listen for the next invitation, a life that knows there were no accidents along the way and none will follow me into the future.

My certainty that the divine has always been the creator of the appointments I have been inclined to make and keep has, in its way, given me the confidence coupled with the willingness to breathe, pause, and breathe again at this time, at this age, with these people who share my journey. Life is a long time from being over, but it's also mandatory, from my current perspective, to take the time to breathe, pause, and breathe again while the mood is still calling me. Can you allow it to call to you too?

A pause is a suspension of activity, a time of temporary disengagement when we are no longer moving toward any goal . . .

—Tara Brach

Right now, before reading any further, take a few moments to yourself to breathe, pause, and breathe again. Sit alone in a room that comforts you. Sit quietly. Close your eyes. Enjoy the moment.

1. Upon "awaking" from this silence, what thoughts come first to mind? Share these thoughts in your journal.
2. What most pleases you about this exercise? Share this thought in your journal too.
3. Will you set aside time to repeat this tomorrow? Why or why not?

1

Step Aside and Experience a Miracle in the Making

I began the practice of "stepping aside" only after years of stepping into business that was clearly not my own. I had mistakenly assumed that helping others make their decisions was an important calling. It showed them I cared. It was my way of remaining important to them. Or so I thought . . .

From childhood on, I had virtually always felt on the edge of abandonment. By girlfriends. By boyfriends. By husbands. Thus, I felt the constant pull to live in the middle of everyone else's life. That way they couldn't forget about me. They couldn't go off, leaving me behind, the way Marcia, my best friend in the sixth grade, left me behind when she chose to ride her bike with Mary after school rather than waiting for me to join them. It stung. It happened again and again. And I carried the fear that would continue to define my life well into my thirties.

The joy I experience now, having finally put to rest the fear of abandonment nearly forty years ago, still remains one of the triumphs of my life. Perhaps this seems like a strange triumph, at least one not worth crowing over, but it's huge to someone like me. Someone who simply had no boundaries between herself and everyone else. It wasn't until 1971, in fact, that I even had a glimmering of what I was doing. What I had always done, in fact, in the presence of others.

What jarred me into a new perspective was a passage in a book by a Jesuit priest, John Powell. The book was *Why Am I*

Afraid to Tell You Who I Am? On page thirty-eight of the edition I was reading, a truth rang out, louder than a train whistle. Powell shares a story with the reader about an experience he had while walking in New York City with a good friend. The friend stopped to buy a newspaper from a street-corner vendor, a stop he made daily and one that Powell had observed him make myriad times. The vendor was always gruff and never said thanks for the generous tip his friend always offered him. Powell, in exasperation, finally asked, "Why do you give him a tip? He is not worthy of one. He is rude to you." His friend quietly replied, "Why should I let him decide what kind of day I am going to have?"

I knew, instantly, this explanation was the key that I could use to unlock the shuttered house I had lived in for so many years. I still remember the awareness I had, as though it was yesterday, that my life could change immediately if I utilized this nugget of information as a guideline for my own relationships. However, we often have to hear a message many times before we can actually adopt it as a tool we can apply to situations that we experience. The seed had been planted, nonetheless. Although it lay dormant for years, it was never forgotten. Never.

Dancing around the many others in my life, seeking both attention and any opportunity to choreograph the experience for all who were present, was my life's work. Or so I thought. Allowing others to create their own dance was far too frightening for me. What if they selected a partner other than me?

Living like this constricted me, of course. It prevented me from discovering the very specific elements of my personal journey, a journey that was significant (as are all journeys), unique, and a divine complement to the journeys of the "chosen" others I met on my path. But trying to force what I wanted my divine plan to be was unsuccessful, of course. Highly unsuccessful. Fortunately. What was, and remains to be, my journey will always call me forth. If I fall back into the pattern I had so painstakingly crafted in the first few decades of my life, I will cease to grow, to understand, to cultivate the seeds that remain within that want me to move to the next level of Karenhood.

Before you think my life is stalemated, or yours too, if what I've shared here has a familiar ring to you—it's not. Far from it, in fact. And that's because I was introduced to a concept I had heretofore neither known nor applied: detachment. Detachment was first explained to me in Al-Anon, a program that I continue to cherish. My ability to use detachment in my life was rife with ample starts but unfortunately with more frequent stops. Detachment was illusive. It slipped through my fingers with ease. A sense of freedom was the reward, however, whenever I successfully detached, stood aside, when the drama that was unfolding before my eyes clearly didn't need my input.

Now, stepping aside is a tool, a truly practical tool that I simply never leave in the toolbox. It's by my side 24/7. It's applied 24/7 too. You may be wondering what stepping aside looks like. It looks like peace. It feels like peace. It initiates peace. It is utilizing the innate ability to observe a situation rather than getting personally involved. It's knowing and practicing how to stay out of the personal business of others. It's being able to remain in a state of relaxation when everyone around you is adding to the drama of the moment. It's staying quiet inside and reflecting the relief that's felt when we know we have just avoided a pitfall that used to snag us every time but no more.

Being able to joyfully look toward our remaining years, knowing they are destined to be as peaceful as we make up our minds they will be, puts us comfortably in the driver's seat for making sure the journey we are celebrating is one that enhances not only ourselves and those close to us, but also every member of the human community, here and on the other side of the globe. How we live in one instant is communicated throughout the cosmos. No doubt about it. Are you ready to take on the charge of helping others, worldwide, to live more peacefully? Then step aside when the drama unfolding before you wears someone else's name. The peace you will feel will mindfully transport you to a place you'll never want to leave. Never ever.

Let me not take to myself, and suffer over, the actions and reactions of other people. Other adult human beings are not my responsibility, no matter how closely their lives may be intertwined with mine.

—One Day at a Time in Al-Anon

———————

Before proceeding on to the next essay, the next shift in thinking, let's stop, truly pause, and breathe in this idea if it's new to you. See and feel how stepping aside when a friend or family member is trying to engage you in a drama you want no part of relieves you of anxiety. In fact, recall when you have tried this most recently, if you have an example. Journal about how that felt.

If you don't have an example, take a moment here to recall a situation during which it would have been perfect for you to step aside, but you got right in there instead. What was that outcome? Journal about that situation. Make a plan for what you might do next time and write it down. Now close your eyes and envision yourself having a successful experience of stepping aside.

Job well done. Go forth now and spread peace.

———————

Hear the Silence, Rest the Mind, Let God Speak

Being at one with the quiet spaces within gently clears the mind, allows the solution to a nagging problem to surface, and draws us close to God and one another. In that closeness, our healing lies. All our answers reside there too. We simply need do nothing to initiate the healing we seek. The healing everyone seeks. It waits for us. It waits for all of us. And when we are ready, it will come. It will come freely.

When I first learned that we need do nothing, that most of what ailed me—ailed all of us, in fact—was rooted in the insatiable ego, I breathed easier. I still didn't understand how things would change, but I did breathe easier. I had always assumed I needed to be busy acquiring information, money, lovers, degrees, friends, accolades. To be at rest, to trust that what I needed to do would present itself to me when the time was right, was unfathomable. I know I'm not alone in this assumption. I believe that what's true for me is true for all of us. Quit chasing. Sit a while. Hear the silence. It will speak to us. Maybe not the first time you and I sit quietly, but as we cultivate the joy of silence, that which we seek will come.

One of the marvelous prizes that comes with aging is that we do have more time, time that seems even more precious now that we are on the "backside of life," to sit quietly in our favorite comfy chair, or on the deck overlooking a garden or a lake, or in a nearby park. We have time to contemplate the stillness. No one can rush us anymore, unless we allow it. We choose the activities we want to experience. Sitting quietly is one of the sweetest ones to call to us.

Wherever you are sitting right now reading this, let's try a tiny experiment. Lay the book aside. Put your feet flat on the floor. If it's comfortable, close your eyes, but not until your hands are resting in your lap. Listen to the quiet all around you. Feel your chest rising with each breath. Notice the images that pass through your mind. With very quiet lips, blow the images away. Absorb the emptiness. When another image comes, blow it away too. Because you can, sit still for the next few minutes. Voice a quiet request to God: "How can I be of help before this day ends?" Sit a spell longer, then open your eyes slowly. Now, trust that what moves your way is your opportunity to offer help. Don't judge it. Simply do what feels right and natural.

Perhaps it seems that life can't be this simple. But it can. No one is watching over your shoulder. We are free to simply be. The years of spinning our wheels are over. Many would say we didn't ever have to spin them even when we did, but we did that which we saw others do. Now we can be the trendsetters. Now we can show others a new way to be. A quiet way to be. A way that promises the rich reward of experiencing the present moment. Only in the present moment can we be healed from the wounds of old. Only in the present moment can we sense God. Only in the present moment can we know our next "suggestion," the assignment that will invite another soul into the experience of healing that we have found. In the stillness that we cultivated are the only suggestions we need to follow.

Amen. Amen.

If a man would travel far along the mystic road, he must learn to desire God intensely but in stillness, passively and yet with all his heart and mind and strength.

—Aldous Huxley

Let's consider some truths before moving ahead:

1. The desire to know God is required to experience God.
2. The wish to experience stillness requires that we let our mind step away from chaos for a spell.
3. Our woundedness is a pathway to seeking connection with others.
4. Our woundedness is our opportunity to experience forgiveness.
5. Breathing freely is our birthright.
6. Experiencing peace is a decision.
7. Teaching others is *the number one fact* of our life. It's happening every moment.
8. Teach only love.

What next?

Listen. Love. Pray. Forgive. And then forgive again.

Go forth today with this thought: I will act from the place of love in my heart. Again and again.

At day's end, make a note in your journal describing your interactions.

What pleased you?

What will you change before going forth tomorrow?

A Faith-Filled Life

Faith is not about everything turning out okay. It's about being okay, no matter how everything turns out.

—Anonymous

I didn't grow up in a faith-filled home. I never observed anyone at 827 being quietly peaceful, trusting that the experiences we were sharing would work out okay. The days and nights were generally very tense, undergirded with the expectation that an outburst over something, large or small, imagined even, might occur at any moment. And usually did. Night after night, the feeling present at the supper table mimicked the feeling at lunch. Tension was served and felt with each bite. Our family doctor, Dr. Cole, told my mother that I had a nervous stomach. What I really had was extreme anxiety that made eating nearly impossible some nights. Living in my home was hard. Peace was something I could never have defined. Tension was all I knew. Tension defined all six of us.

I did have a place I loved to be, though, and that was in Logansport with my grandparents. My grandmother had a quiet presence about her. No wonder I loved to visit them. Her comforting words and arms and smiles would temporarily convince me that everything was okay. When I thought about home when I was with her, my stomach would twist and turn. I hated to feel, even from afar, the tension at home. I feared it would never change. And as a matter of fact, it never did. Not even with the passage of time. Tension was as fresh in my parents' old age as when they were young. How tragic, really.

Tension is hard on all of us. No matter our age. But we choose the feeling, as strange as that may seem. Unfortunately, we seldom understand how and when we made that choice. Certainly I didn't know I had chosen it. We do imitate that which we observe, however. And my times with my grandmother were simply too short for me to adapt to her way of living and seeing the world.

For many who grew up in environments like mine, leaving home, choosing to be surrounded by new philosophies, new people, new opportunities, became necessary in order to catch a glimpse of a life free from tension. And that glimpse didn't come very quickly for me. It took a few years, a few bad relationships, one painful marriage, and multiple suicide considerations before I was solidly awakened to a better choice, a saner perspective, a softer, kinder feeling within. What brought me to this new experience of faith, this place of wellbeing, was two decades of near constant alcohol and drug use that could have ended my life. But I reached that new place. I arrived at a saner, faith-filled place with the help of friends who had been sent to make sure I'd arrive. The place had a name; it was called Alcoholics Anonymous.

I don't mean to suggest that anyone else needs to travel my path to find faith, to reach that peaceful place of knowing that everything is okay. But that's what I had to do. We can get here following any number of paths. There is no right one. The goal is just to seek a path until you find it, then travel it, share what you know if someone expresses an interest, model faith for others without making a point of it, and give it away when you can so that it can be kept. Having faith is like having the gold ring in your pocket that you grabbed on the merry-go-round when you were a child. That ring promised you another ride whenever you wanted to claim it. Like faith, it would always be there. And even when you used it, you knew another gold ring was yours for the taking.

It's funny, really; I don't even ponder my faith any longer. I simply live it. I never doubt that God is present, that all is well, that what I need to experience will come calling, that who I need to meet might be around the next bend in the road. Even when I don't like what might be happening, I know that what is happening is the next right experience for me. My faith has taught me that. Again and again. And life feels simple and calm and intentional. Most of all, it feels purposeful. I do what's on the chart for me, and God is pleased. This I believe.

Are you at peace?

Has your life measured up in the way you had hoped it would?

Do you long for a more faith-filled life?

It's not too late to create it. Here are some suggestions that I can vouch for. Maybe one or two will appeal to you:

1. Make a list of what you are grateful for in your life. How has each one made you a better person?
2. Make a practice of having a short conversation with God each morning, either right before your feet hit the floor or right after.
3. Ask him for his help in everything you are called on to do.
4. Be prepared to thank God throughout the day for all of the little miracles that seem to be happening, miracles you might not have noticed before.
5. Be ready and willing to help the first person you meet. At the very least, greet him or her with a smile.

6. And if you are still failing to connect with God, write him a note and ask for help.
7. Share with your closest friend a few of the events in your life when God "showed up."
8. Keep a list of these special experiences close at hand for those times that you doubt his availability.

Now relax. God is in charge and he doesn't need your help today.

_____

4

Rapt Attention

Rapt attention is the greatest gift we can give to one another, to the natural world around us, to all that's seen and not seen but only felt. Being fully present to all is how we acknowledge and honor God.

At least thirty-five years ago, my husband, an artist who works in many media, created a beautiful eight-foot cross that was to be carried by the priests at St. Stephen's Church in their ceremonial processionals. He asked me if I could think of a good quote to embed in the base of the cross, and I suggested: "Rapt attention is the greatest gift we can give to one another." I continue to believe it is the greatest gift.

One of the beauties of this gift is its simplicity. We don't need any special qualities to do it. We need nothing more than desire. And then the willingness to bestow our attention on whoever stands before us, knowing that he or she has been summoned by the Spirit within, unabashedly summoned.

I haven't always been comfortable with the idea that I, that we, summon whoever comes to greet us. All those "greeters" have one thing in common: they serve as teachers within the curriculum we have designed. But with Caroline Myss's help, I grew to trust the idea. Myss is a spiritual intuitive who has written many books, including *Sacred Contracts: Awakening Your Divine Potential*. That book moved me to my acceptance of the idea, an idea that has been more transformative than any singular idea I have ever been introduced to: *not one person* who has ever signaled to me, who has ever boldly or quietly caught my attention, was on my radar screen willy-nilly. And with my acceptance of that came profound awe.

Perhaps you are doubtful of the veracity of this idea. I certainly was when I first heard it. And even after I had inched closer to believing it, I still had reservations. How could the one who had abused me at such a young age have been summoned by me? Myss's explanation was that we "designed" our lessons, and "our partners" agreed to be part of our learning. There was no judgment, good or bad, attached to the lessons. They simply were the experiences that defined our lives, in the process making us more whole, more spiritual, more necessary to the remaining people we'd meet and learn to love.

Before going a step further, close your eyes and remember one of your "lessons" that has helped you be who you are today. In your journal, share what you realize now was the specific enhancement to your life that resulted from the experience. Do you now relish the lesson in spite of how it no doubt looked and felt at the time of the teaching?

Forgiveness was my lesson. A profound expression of forgiveness that only came after I was drawn to offer it to the perpetrator of my abuse in the silence of my mind. I'm relieved to tell you that my life never felt the same once I got to the big "payoff." The willingness to forgive was the first step, of course. The forgiveness, itself, is what transformed me, and I believe it is what transforms all of us.

You may be wondering how this story of mine relates to rapt attention, what I consider to be our greatest gift. Here is how I see it. The perpetrator, in a sense, demanded my attention because of the experience itself. But then what remained for years in my mind was the shadow of the experience, always taking away from the attention that the person standing before me deserved.

My introduction to Myss and her theory about all of the people who make the journey with us jarringly established that *he, too,* had been a necessary part of my journey. When I sought to understand why such an invasive lesson was necessary, I was shown that forgiveness, one of the hardest of all human challenges, when fully practiced, changes us profoundly in all the right ways. It transforms us into the people who can eventually heal others by our example. And that oftentimes it demands harsh experiences to elicit its full impact.

I know I was forever changed. And the rapt attention everyone is deserving of can now be expressed. Completely. Do I give that attention always? Of course not. Life is a series of missteps. But I still have the last quarter of life to practice in. The last quarter. Sounds a bit ominous. But that's all in the choice. I can see it as the best quarter of all because my worries are few. And you? You can make this choice too.

Your most important lesson: What was it? How have you grown from it?

What does the concept of rapt attention mean to you? Is it a gift that you bestow freely on others?

1. Share about these two ideas in your journal.
2. Tell a friend why he or she is important to you. It's an exercise that will have a profound impact on your relationship. And on your inner child too.
3. It's never too late to change how we look at our lives, our friends, the strangers who cross our paths, the many we barely noticed in years gone by. They too had messages.
4. Someone will still try to reach you with a message you need. Be alert!

5

Say Something Kind or Nothing at All

Mother Teresa says be kind to everyone, and start with the person standing next to you. I love the simplicity of that suggestion. Don't you? We aren't asked to evaluate anything about the person. Her dress, his fingernails, the frown or the easy smile. The sound of her voice isn't the determiner of our reaction. Nor is what he says to us or to anyone else. Very simply, just be kind. No matter what.

As I age, I appreciate Mother Teresa's words even more. I think we all want meaningful lives. We all want to look back as well as forward with a sense of peace about how we have lived and how we intend to live as the days ahead turn into weeks and years. Regrets? Of course I have some. But they will be fewer if I apply Mother Teresa's tiny suggestion.

This suggestion also reminds me of what mothers used to tell us as children: "If you can't say something nice about someone, don't say anything at all." Kindergarten logic, it was called. But it was wise beyond measure, I think. Adopting this philosophy as one's guidepost for living will have a major impact not only on your own sense of wellbeing and what you can contribute to the others in your circle, but also on men and women, children and young adults around the globe. What we do in one place with one person has a ripple effect that knows no end. Seem farfetched? Not at all. Some scientists call it the "butterfly effect." I love the truth of it. It means we are helping, or hurting all others everywhere with every action we take. Making the decision to be kind, simply kind, always, is one way each of us can add benefit to the world we share. Why not give it a try?

In order to make good use of Mother Teresa's suggestion, let's inventory our actions of late, and then monitor them in the future for a period of time. Why? That's the only sound way we can be certain we are becoming the people we'd rather be. Now I don't want to push you into a corner, so if this exercise doesn't appeal to you, at least not at the present time, that's okay. Move on to another essay and discover how it might speak to you. But I'm inclined to think that many of us really do want to change how we respond to the people around us. And because treating one person well actually treats many people well, it's a simple way to make a very important contribution to the human community.

Looking at the recent past:

1. What instances can you recall when you could have shown a kinder hand to the people or person you were having an exchange with? If you were to re-experience that encounter, how would you prefer showing up? Take a moment to write about it in your journal. We make changes more easily when we put them in writing.

2. Please share those times when you could have celebrated how you behaved. What feedback did you receive from the person or people involved? What has it taught you about your future?

3. Being who we want to be is little more than a decision. The decision to be kind is really an easy one to make. And it relieves us of all stress. We know, without even thinking about it, what we will do in every encounter. *Every one.*

6

The Journey Is Perfect, the Stumbles as Well as the Strides

I don't know about you, but I have stumbled many times getting to where I am now. I began stumbling, literally, when I took my first drink at thirteen. Hiding behind the garage at an outdoor family gathering, I gulped down my whiskey and coke before anyone could notice me. The rush I felt was quickly matched by the uneasiness I experienced as I headed back to the group. With darting vision, I hurried into the house so no one would guess what I had been up to.

What I could have learned then was that alcohol had the capacity to trip a person up in more ways than one. However, what I learned instead over the next few months was that with every drink I took, I felt a bit less fear. Around boys in particular. Over time, the continued use of alcohol gave me the courage to stand apart, to move forward, even to eventually set many highfalutin goals, most of which seemed way beyond my reach, throughout the next thirty-three years.

As an example, I'm convinced that I would not have tackled graduate school following the demise of my twelve-year marriage if I had not *fueled up* on alcohol. Perhaps that seems like a farfetched idea, but I'd venture to guess that many alcoholics in the rooms of AA would concur. We could muffle the cries of the scared ego if we drank just one more whiskey on ice. I knew I wasn't a scholar, in my sober moments; but with a little alcohol in my system, I was certain I could accomplish what the others around me were accomplishing. And one of the areas I was fearless about was writing. While I observed my fellow students avoiding like the plague the major papers that were required for every course, I eagerly leapt to the challenge. Unafraid. Undaunted. Undeterred.

That I met the challenge successfully gave structure to the rest of my life. Learning, as I did, how pleasurable writing could be set the stage for my passion to flourish. Twenty-nine books later and I'm still committed to the dream. The fortunate news is that I didn't have to keep drinking to accomplish it. In fact, had I continued to drink, I would have failed the final test. Writing the dissertation took a sober head. I feared I couldn't master that. But I did, with the help of many others.

I am not assuming that you, the reader, had a journey like mine, one that was both helped and then hindered by alcohol, but before I go further, let's pause. Think about your own journey from your teen years to now. Just close your eyes for a few minutes. Just as suggested in the introduction, pause, breathe, and pause again.

What do you see and feel?

What could have deterred your journey but didn't? Or if it did, for a spell, what happened to change your course? To pull you back on track?

Does it seem to you that your trajectory has been intentional? What does that mean, in fact?

I am comforted by the opinion that our journeys are quite intentional. That they were predetermined; some would say preordained. Caroline Myss, the spiritual intuitive I referred to earlier, says that all experiences with all others are "sacred contracts," encounters agreed to before "awakening" into this life we currently lead. She says the agreements we made are equivalent to the "education" we receive. And that education is not only for our benefit, but for the benefit of others as well.

I am well aware of how some of my experiences strengthened my character and served as the example to others of what a single experience is capable of doing for us. For instance, as I mentioned in another essay, I learned the true depth of forgiveness as a result of an unwanted sexual encounter when I was a young girl. It was not sought by me, of course. I was an unwitting participant, and I was haunted by the many experiences for decades thereafter. Had I had an inkling that I was going to be privy to the real meaning of forgiveness as a result of the encounters, perhaps I would not have been so frightened by them. But I didn't know. I didn't understand. I didn't see the big spiritual picture. And it wasn't until I read Myss's *Sacred Contracts* that I fully understood the meaning behind the experiences, a meaning that has informed my life like no other:

You probably know people who seem to have had their entire life mapped out from the day they were born. You may have envied their sure sense of what they were born to do—their work, career, marriage, and personal goals.

And yet you have probably also wondered whether that was really all there was to it. So have I. The answer I found is that there's much more involved. I believe that each of us is guided by a Sacred Contract that our soul made before we were born. That Contract contains a wide range of agreements regarding all that we are intended to learn in this life. It comprises not merely what kind of work we do but also our key relationships with the people who are to help us learn the lessons we have agreed to work on. Each of those relationships represents an individual Contract that is part of

your overall Sacred Contract, and may require you to be in a certain place at a certain time to be with that person.

—Caroline Myss, Myss Library

Before moving on to another essay, can you see an overall pattern to your life? If so, name as many features as you can.

What surprises you most about your life now?

What pleases you the most?

7

Fear and Anger

Any expression that is not loving is a call for healing and help that is initiated by fear.

—*A Course in Miracles*

More than thirty years ago, I was introduced to *A Course in Miracles*. Although initially resistant to it, I slowly took it in and discovered that it satisfied my yearning for an additional spiritual pathway, one that complemented my 12-step journey. One of its primary concepts astounded me: any expression, verbal or physical, that isn't loving has been triggered by fear and it's simply a call for help. More important, after allowing time to absorb the idea, one that was indeed foreign to me, it completely shifted my perspective. This, in turn, opened my heart. It felt like I was seeing for the first time. Seeing members of my family, in particular my dad, in a way I had never seen them before. To see my father as a fear-filled man, rather than a rage-filled man, made a huge difference to me. I no longer had to rage back at him. I no longer had to sit in judgment.

Accepting my dad, and other angry people too, as fearful rather than rageful meant I could quietly step aside and let them be. Simply let them be. And then, adopting another of the course's principles, I could decide to love them anyway, all of them. Meeting fear/anger with an expression of love is the shift that little by little changes the universe we share with seven billion other souls. Little by little, each expression of love roots out festering rage. Little by little, the world we'd rather live in becomes manifest, at least within our own small circle.

Let's pause here and think about our own recent past. Perhaps it would help to enumerate the times in this last week when you either felt anger, or observed someone else expressing anger, perhaps a friend or a family member. What were the circumstances and who were the players?

List them in your journal. Can you guess what caused the anger? Can you see where fear had a role to play? What did the fear look like? If you were directly involved in the experience, consider reliving the experience, except this time willingly expressing love and acceptance of the person or the situation.

How does it feel? How does love and acceptance change the tenor of the moment and impact those present? Share your observations before going on. This is a learning opportunity.

If queried by the others present, what will you tell them about the concept of love versus fear?

I have found that it simplifies my life to categorize, as either love or fear, the actions and expressions of the people I live among. When I, in turn, express only love, regardless of what I have experienced from those around me, I feel free. I feel filled with hope. I feel a contentment about the future that eases every moment of anticipation. Having the capacity and willingness to live this way has changed every moment of my life. I spent much of the first half of my life in near-constant dread of what would befall me next. Fear ruled my life. Thus I was quick to anger, just as my dad had been. But that's the past. My present is far different from my past.

What does your present look like?

Do you go into your experiences with a sense of wellbeing?

In what situations, in particular, do you wish you could "show up" differently?

There is a way to do it. Begin by taking a deep breath. Envision yourself being the better you within a particular circumstance. Play it all the way through to the end. Just rest in this arena for a spell.

What is going on within you now?

Would you like to live here permanently? It's your choice. It's always your choice. All it demands of you is a statement of purpose followed by an internal decision.

Let's cherish the new you.

8

Change Is Good

When we are no longer able to change a situation, we are challenged to change ourselves.

—Viktor E. Frankl

Change is an interesting opportunity. Perhaps you haven't thought about it in that way. Resisting change is generally the more common response. But let's take the next few minutes and list in our journals a few of the changes we have experienced in the last decade.

Are there any similarities in the kinds of changes?

Which one of the above changes was easiest to undergo? Can you guess why?

Which one has "paid off" the most?

What I am trying to get across is that change is good. Change is intentional. It never comes our way unless we are prepared for it. We may not realize we are ready for the change, but no change visits us that we have not been readied for. Absolutely none. How can I be so sure? Remember the *Sacred Contracts* that we discussed in two earlier essays? Whatever crosses your path has been invited. Whoever is present is a chosen guest, one with a lesson for you. Wherever you are is the perfect location. There are no coincidences. None!

Now revisit the "dreaded" changes you were forced to make at an earlier time in your life. If it helps to close your eyes, do so.

What were you thinking in the midst of the change? Can you remember what it felt like to make the necessary adjustment? It was a door opener. Change always is. Let's savor the new ideas we were introduced to, and the new people too. Share here your overriding feeling after the adjustment was made.

What's the best holdover from that originally unexpected and dreaded change? How has it benefitted your life?

Have you been able to transfer some of the benefit to the lives of others? Hopefully you can see how that has happened. Nothing ever happens in our experience that doesn't have a broader use. Trace that use now and be pleased you were the conduit for change in others.

Perhaps you are still resisting change rather than celebrating the idea that you are ready for new growth, or change would not have come knocking. The aging process introduces all of us to many changes. I certainly see many in my life. Appearance, flexibility, eyesight, and wrinkles, to name just a few. But there's also peace of mind. Acceptance of what I can't change. And greater joy over the small things in life. It's actually time to celebrate who we were, who we are, and celebrate the possibilities for the future. Share here what you are currently celebrating.

9

What's Next?

Though no one can go back and make a brand new start, anyone can start from now and make a brand new ending.

—Carl Bard

What do we do now that life as we knew it is over? What do we do now that no one is waiting for us to kick off the early morning meeting? Is there a place to hang our hat, so to speak? Is there any place we are needed? Or are we finished, simply finished? Not at all.

These are good questions, I think, for us to consider as we round this corner of life. The big job has been packed away. Now we are searching for activities that will keep us vibrant, engaged, fulfilled, and happy. "Most folks are as happy as they make up their minds to be," says Abraham Lincoln. Activities that offer all four (vibrancy, engagement, fulfillment, and happiness) are often intensely focused on the lives of others; usually others who have been bombarded by difficulties. The opportunities to volunteer to make a difference in the lives of people in your community are many. And too often the response to these opportunities is negligible.

Perhaps you are wondering why an essay on this topic is here in this book, a book that focuses on the rest of our journey. But the answer should be obvious. For many, the journey to this stage of life has been meaningful, profitable, and fulfilling. The fear about getting out of bed on day one of the next stage of life will be traumatic for some, because there is no office to go to, no letters to dictate, no meetings to hold, no advice to be offered. The connection to others was the glue that enriched our lives, but many never realized that involvement with others was the key that opened the door to one's heart. But it was. The heart is waiting to be opened again. So don't tarry in the "what's next?" stage too long.

I'm offering this idea to you because so much remains to be done to make life even tolerable for millions of people. People in this country, as well as people all over the continent, are living in poverty. Millions are starved for food, medicine, education, clean water, decent housing. I just read an article today about a world food program that is run by a former colleague of mine. It's their goal to ship 240,000,000 meals next year. That's a huge number, but it's a drop in the bucket when we consider there are seven billion people on the planet, and research shows that at least 1.02 billion of them go to bed hungry every day. *Every day.*

If you want to make a difference, and most of us do, look at the listings of volunteer opportunities in your local newspaper or online. Want to help children? Be a tutor or a mentor. Want to help with the elderly or the infirm? Visit a local nursing home and ask what you might do. Contact the food bank in your town and see what help they need. Or the homeless shelter. Or a meals-on-wheels program. If cooking is your thing, see what you can do at a kitchen serving the homeless. The opportunities to help others are many. And any help any one of us gives helps us too. Giving back is what makes our own lives rich and meaningful.

On the evening news, nearly every day the closing story is about a person or family, sometimes even a child, who has extended themselves to make a difference in the lives of others. One of the remarkable things about each person is that they don't feel heroic at all. Their humility is evident. What others do isn't beyond the reach of any of us. Maybe our skills are different, but wherever there's a desire, there is a way to make that difference. And the payback is tenfold. *Tenfold.*

If you are one of those individuals who is trying to figure out what to do now that your life has allowed you so much leisure time, begin by making a list of what you'd want someone to do for you if your circumstances were dire, or even if you were simply lonely. What comes first to mind? A good conversation, perhaps? Someone to simply sit with you as a listener to whatever you want to talk about? How about a friend to take you out for a drive, maybe through the neighborhood of your childhood? Or to go for a meal with you at one of your favorite restaurants?

Looking through the photos of your past, sharing the back story of the pictures, would be a great gift of time to many. Maybe having someone help you write letters to people you haven't forgotten, or to those you have a fond memory of. Perhaps you have always wanted to take a painting class, but prefer sharing the experience with someone else. Nursing homes or assisted living facilities are no doubt filled with folks who would love to accompany you, making two people happy at the same time.

The ways to continue the interactions that have always made your life rich and rewarding don't end just because you no longer receive a paycheck. Indeed, just the opposite is true. Now you can fulfill your personal passion and draw someone else into your dream at the same time. Witnessing another, while being witnessed, makes for a sacred experience, one not to be lived lightly.

What joy this new part of our journey can bring if we decide to show up for it. Begin a list in your journal of all the things you can imagine doing. Perhaps even some that seem a real stretch for you. Be daring. Be creative. Be *an even better you* than heretofore.

Check in here or elsewhere after you have begun reaching out. How do you see your life changing? What's the most exciting part of the change?

———————————

10

Forgive Yourself Completely

Is there really a need for us to forgive ourselves? Some may think not, and it's an individual decision, certainly. The trajectory of my life, however, has clearly shown me that forgiveness is necessary. I walked myself into many dark alleys; hung out with many questionable men; and straddled the very thin line between barely acceptable and totally unacceptable behavior for more than twenty years, from ages sixteen to thirty-six, when I finally looked at who I had become and got sober. That I lived to tell my story is due to the presence of "hovering angels," I'm convinced. And I'm grateful to be telling the story, rather than having my story told by someone else.

As a child I never considered the possibility that *someone* was watching over me. That idea wasn't ever addressed in my family, around the supper table or at bedtime. Mother didn't lead us in prayer. Nor was grace spoken when we gathered to eat, except on special occasions when Uncle George thumped the Bible hard on behalf of us all. I don't believe my family of six was a godless family, but we didn't claim reliance on God either. I simply never considered his presence. Nor did anyone else, to my knowledge. Praying about a decision I had to make was a very foreign idea. A very foreign idea indeed.

How different my life might have been if I had lived as though God were my daily companion, available for consultation on a regular basis. Many decisions would have been different. Many behaviors never attempted. Many encounters avoided. Many reasons for feeling grateful would have presented themselves. Many actions for which I had to eventually forgive myself would have been sidestepped. The interesting thing, however, is that I believe wholeheartedly that whatever any one of us needs to learn will make its way to us. In time. Absolutely.

Having that belief as one of my treasured truths in these last few decades of living has given me a sense of wellbeing, coupled with the assurance that I will be presented with every experience I need, now and in the years ahead. And because I trust that the God of my understanding will be involved, I'll not be creating unnecessary drama or reasons for self- or other forgiveness. In case this sounds like forgiveness is something we want to avoid, I want to offer assurance that forgiveness is an act of joining with our inner self or with those around us. It's a kind gesture, always. It's honorable, loving, and a symbol of self-acceptance. It's a way of saying to the God of our understanding, "I know you are present, here and now, and I am grateful."

One of the things I have had to undertake, since becoming sober, is to create a list of opportunities for forgiveness, either of myself or someone else. Making the list, in and of itself, is a humbling experience. It's looking at ourselves straight on, with no room for avoidance. It's freeing too, once we have begun the list. Writing down one thing, just one thing, is what removes the barriers to our past.

I had to forgive myself for abusing my body with alcohol and drugs. Alcohol and drugs, coupled with putting myself in harm's way because of the choices I made for companionship, all deserved careful consideration and far more than just a nod of forgiveness. I dangled for many years over the abyss, a choice that I made with eyes opened. That there was a presence watching over me, an unacknowledged one for sure, made it possible for me to eventually get back on track and become the woman I had been charted to be so long ago.

All who are reading this have pasts too, perhaps far different from mine, but there have been experiences that cast shadows,

I'm sure. After all, we are human. We sometimes dodge our responsibilities. Even worse, perhaps we caused harm to others and turned away rather than admitting it. But nothing, nothing was so awful that you and I aren't worthy of forgiveness—from ourselves, from our companions, and from God too. With God, all is forgiven. Always.

––––––––––––

A good exercise for all of us is to take an inventory, however brief, and begin the process of seeing ourselves *as we are*, not how we pretend to be. Dig deep. Look at yourself straight on, not sideways. Be daring. And then get down to the business of forgiveness. If it helps, and I think it will, take pen to paper and write: I forgive you, _____ (put your name here), for this past action, _____ (put what it was here), and now it's time to rejoice. Note the many experiences that come to mind. Don't think anything is too small to write down. If it came to mind, it's worthy of attention.

At another time, begin this process again, forgiving *others* for their transgressions. Only when we are free from our past issues will we face the future with healthy anticipation. Decades of living are behind us now; there is no time to tarry. What lies ahead will be as good as we are willing to allow it to be.

––––––––––––

The truth is, unless you let go, unless you forgive yourself, unless you forgive the situation, unless you realize that the situation is over, you cannot move forward.

—Steve Maraboli

11

Remembrances

Everyone must leave something behind when he dies, my grandfather said. A child or a book or a painting or a house or a wall built or a pair of shoes made. Or a garden planted. Something your hand touched some way so your soul has somewhere to go when you die, and when people look at that tree or that flower you planted, you're there.

—Ray Bradbury

I have lost a number of very good friends over the past couple of years. And I have mementos from three of the women in my study. A rock from one friend, a book from another, and a pin from the third. I find myself looking at their pictures, holding their remembrances, and feeling their presence in a very distinct way each time, just as Bradbury suggests in the above quote.

I think of these women, and my mother too, as the angels who hover around my shoulders at good times, as well as at difficult times. And actually, I have very few difficult times anymore. I'm inclined to think it might be because I have the protection of Joy, Cate, Beverly, and Mom, particularly Mom, who shared a secret with me, one that put closure on an earlier chapter of my life and hers. That secret became the glue that drew us into a relationship so sweet.

Arriving at the threshold of seventy-five, nearly takes my breath away. How could the years have passed so quickly? Death may well be twenty years from now, and I hope it is (if my health holds), but most of my life has already been lived.

Regardless, I remember so well second grade, Miss White and the point of her pencil pushing against my skull. I begged to get out of her classroom. No dice. And I can't forget Mr. Priest and the sixth grade picnic at his cabin on the river. I got the worst sunburn of my life, perhaps because I insisted on wearing the halter top my mother said was too baring. I couldn't stand the feeling of clothes touching my shoulders for days.

And remembering my first bonafide date with Steve, the love of my life in high school, still makes my heart race a bit. Like so many other girls in the '50s, I was sure that if he and I married it would be forever. It was never to be, of course. Most high school romances come to a necessary end.

All things have their end, in one respect. Experiences. People. Sometimes relationships too. I don't mean for this essay to be maudlin. On the contrary, I think that what lies ahead in this life, or the next, will be greater than my heart or mind can currently imagine. I don't think of my loved ones on the other side as shadowy figures. I think of them as still vibrant, just living life in a different form. To some this may seem crazy, but it fills me with joy to remember Joy, her laughter, her sense of humor, the way she had of bringing dark experiences into the light of acceptance. We laughed with her. I still laugh with her when I recall some of her stories. And I have a strong sense that she hears me. I think actively remembering our loved ones who have passed into the next realm keeps them "working" on our behalf. And I, for one, figure I need all the help I can get.

What are your thoughts about dying or the dead who have passed already? You have some, for sure. Perhaps no one has so pointedly asked you this before, but digging deep to reveal our inner thoughts in this latter stage of life is good for us. I'm sure of it. Do you consider the dead as helpmates for your journey here? I like the belief that our opportunities to help others and be helped, in return, never end. If Bradbury is right, and the spirit of each of us is left within an item we can see or touch, it suggests the sacred presence of any one of us is present with every one of us for all time. What a delicious thought.

Whom do you remember dearly? And why?

And whom do you hope will keep your spirit alive? Why?

Journaling a while about these questions will clarify what you believe, thus revealing to you some opportunities for new directions. Check out the family pictures, see who is there and wants to be remembered. Note an item on your desk or in a drawer or on a bookshelf that might have come from a loved one that is no longer here in the flesh.

What does this item tell you?

Why have you hung on to it?

What have you passed on to a loved one that he or she may cherish?

What did the item mean to you?

What do you hope it means to her or him?

What is it about eternity that appeals to you? Or not?

As Edwin Hubbell Chapin said, "Every action in our lives touches on some chord that will vibrate in eternity." What a sweet thought to cherish.

12

I Can Choose Peace Instead of This

I've mentioned in other essays how important *A Course in Miracles* has been to my spiritual development. Because the course complements the twelve steps of AA and Al-Anon, I feel many moments of actual joy nearly every day, a payoff I had never expected. These three pathways have grounded me. For sure, had I not found both 12-step programs a number of decades ago, prior to my introduction to the course, I wouldn't be alive to explore the ideas I'm tossing your way here. I was headed down a very dark alley, completely unaware of how dire my circumstances were, absolutely ignorant of the danger of my chosen journey then, and without a doubt, hellbent on being my own worst enemy.

Perhaps some of you can relate. A book such as this probably wouldn't have drawn you in if you had never traveled the rocky roads of life. But then, who doesn't end up on a rocky road, at least occasionally? Rocky roads give rise to our lessons. And the lessons are why we live. It's a cycle, though not a vicious one. It just is what it is.

The title of this essay is "I can choose peace instead of this . . ." You might be wondering what that means. Here's my take: no one is in charge of my thoughts but me. *No one!* No one is in charge of my actions either. I can and will "show up" however I choose, every instant, within every encounter, whether with a friend, a colleague, a family member, or a stranger. Knowing that we have the power, the total power to decide who we will be every instant, makes choosing to be peaceful, rather than controlled by the ugliness of others, a delicious choice. Our choice serves as a great role model for others too. Without suggesting to anyone that they should also choose peace, they see *our reward* for themselves. Actions can speak far louder than words.

When I choose to sit on the sidelines, watching a drama rather than trying to manage it, particularly one that doesn't concern me, my heart isn't elevated. My mind doesn't race. I don't feel nervous, or breathless, or emotional. I experience a sense of warm, loving detachment and know immediately that I want more of that feeling. And now I know where to get it. I can and will feel peace, instead of whatever might have nabbed my emotions, when I stay in charge of what I want to feel, say, and do. This peace is available to you as well.

Enough about my feelings, my choices, and my development. It's time to explore who you are, what you feel, how you choose what you will do or say or think or feel in the myriad circumstances that fly in your direction. Let's pause before beginning the next step.

Is there anything we have talked about here that you'd like to share with a spouse or a friend? I hope so. Let's move forward together. All of us. But before doing so, write a note to a loved one about what you have learned from this particular essay. In this way, you will improve your own chances of repeating the choice in the future and you will have added benefit to your friend's life and to the lives of everyone on this planet. What we do to one, we do to all. It's called the butterfly effect. We will talk more about this in later essays.

Additionally, enriching this latter stage of life in any way we can for ourselves and others is a gift beyond measure. I promise you this.

What do you do when you take a time out from the activities that call to you? Do you meditate? If yes, do so now. If not, just close your eyes and seek to become aware of your breathing for the next few minutes.

1. What's the most recent time you felt agitation? Can you honestly assess whether you were sticking your nose into something that didn't concern you? If yes, let's revisit this scenario in your mind and choose another response to the situation. Write about this experience, the before and after of making a new choice. Focus on how a different choice made you feel.

2. Can you come up with three times in the last week that "choosing peace instead of this . . ." might have been valuable? Write about them here. It's to make an indelible impression on you that I'm suggesting this.

3. Even though taking another person's inventory isn't our business, it's helpful to take note of when others have overstepped their bounds too. Can you think of a few instances? Share those here, not as a way to judge yourself superior, but so you can get better at recognizing your own and others' interference in matters not their/your own.

4. What do you appreciate the most about choosing peace over any other kind of response, now that you have had some time to consider this? Do you imagine you will make peace a more conscious choice in the future?

5. How are you feeling right now?

13

An Inventory

It is said that if we don't learn from our history, we will repeat it. This is true on the world stage and for us as individuals, I think. Let's take an inventory of our lives and check this out.

Probably everyone reading this essay has made a lot of mistakes over the years. Life isn't always pretty, at least mine wasn't. It's not expected to be, in fact, but far too many of us never quit blaming ourselves for mistakes of the past. For some of us, every mistake felt like a tragedy of epic proportions, even when that wasn't the case. And most often it wasn't the case. Many mistakes were simply pebbles on the learning curve of life. Pebbles that might have tripped us, but certainly not big enough pebbles to throw our entire life into a shadow that haunts us into old age.

I know I let folks down in the past, my parents in particular. And even though I made amends, both verbally and by changing my behavior quite dramatically, I still have moments of remorse for the embarrassment I caused them. I think this is partly due to my age now. As I have gotten older, I feel more deeply about what good people they were and know they didn't deserve what I put them through. Excusing it by saying I was simply having growing pains doesn't seem to be enough most of the time. And yet, to continue holding myself hostage means I am missing out on opportunities that are presenting themselves to me every day, opportunities to make a difference in the here and now in the lives of those God is intentionally sending my way.

Whatever your age right now, it's time to move on. It's time to say we have passed through many stages of life, some more successfully than others, but in each stage we met those individuals we were meant to meet. We were introduced to the lessons we were meant to experience. And anything we failed to learn will revisit us at another time. Nothing goes unlearned! Nothing.

Perhaps we should begin here making a list of those things we know we have learned and need no reminders about. Let me name a few so you can get the idea.

1. I have learned that fear wears many faces and one of them is anger.

2. I have learned that letting other people be in charge of their own journey through life is the only way to ensure my peace of mind.

3. I have learned that multitasking is a myth. I can't give my full attention to two places or people at the same time, and each situation is deserving of my rapt, unyielding attention, or it wouldn't have presented itself to me.

4. I have learned that no experience was unimportant to my evolution.

5. I have learned that every expression made by any one of us reflects a feeling of love or fear, and the right response, regardless of what we encounter, is always a loving one. Always.

6. I have learned that we are always in the right place at the right time. Even when it seems this can't possibly be true, it is.

7. I have learned that forgiveness is the only act that truly unifies us, and the acceptance that we are all one is the singular fact of this life we share with seven billion other souls.

8. I have learned that a peaceful heart is the by-product of acting in a peaceful way.

9. I have learned that pausing before making any comment or taking any action is all the time God needs to get the right thought in my mind.

10. I have learned that accepting every encounter with anyone, as holy and part of my divine journey, keeps all chaos at bay.

11. I have learned that I don't have to believe in God for God to believe in me.

Now it's your turn. What do you know to be true?

What do you hope to believe for this last phase of your life?

What's the first thing you plan to do to expand your awareness of God's presence?

14

The Purpose of Life Is to Be Happy

I believe that the very purpose of life is to be happy. From the very core of our being, we desire contentment. In my own limited experience I have found that the more we care for the happiness of others, the greater is our own sense of wellbeing.

—Dalai Lama

I surely couldn't have expressed any more clearly the sentiment shared by the Dalai Lama in the above quote. We too often think our purpose in life needs to be far grander than to just usher in a few happy moments in another person's life. If we can create, for just one person, an hour or a moment of genuine peace and wellbeing, we will have lived a worthy life. His words remind me of Mother Teresa's when she said so simply, "Be kind to everyone and start with the person standing next to you."

Don't misunderstand. We need the superstars too—the Bill Gateses and the Warren Buffets. We need the Hillary Clintons and the Bill O'Reillys. The Jon Stewarts and the Oprah Winfreys. People who reach from afar into our lives and make us think; they make us take a stand; they make us better people. But not everyone needs such a public persona. If you and I simply make a tiny positive difference in the life of one person a day, the kind of difference that makes a person know she or he has been seen and heard, we will have done our job. We will have moved the gauge marking universal peace one notch closer to being accomplished. And that's a mighty accomplishment, indeed.

That's helping humankind move closer to the critical mass that's necessary for all harsh attitudes, all unnecessary wars and even minor strife to be over, once and for all.

Assuredly we can all remember being asked when we were youngsters, "What are you going to be when you grow up?" And had we answered, "Make someone happy," the questioner would likely have scoffed. That answer would not have demonstrated a lofty enough dream. It would not have shown a commitment to personal success. But it might have served the universe in a far better way. *Far better*. Reaching into the life of someone close by and paying heed to their existence is a gift like no other.

Perhaps you are thinking this is simply not doing enough for humankind. Perhaps you are wondering how an activity so simple, so common, can put food on the table and a roof over one's head. My point is not that work that draws a paycheck isn't valuable. Of course it is, but judging one's success by the size of one's paycheck or one's portfolio is missing the point of personal worth. The Mother Teresas of the world measure worth by the smallest of deeds we do for one another. And one of the smallest is the gentle smile. Just a gentle, sincere smile.

Perhaps you are reading this and thinking there has to be more. Perhaps you can't shake the dogma you were fed in your youth regarding success: how it looked, what it meant, why only certain standards counted as real measures of success. And you are reading this and wondering, *Who is this Karen Casey to tell me that none of that mattered?* Don't misunderstand. Please. Any work we did, or continue to do, counted. But the smallest token of appreciation for another's presence on one's journey is what really matters, and that act requires little more than willingness. It doesn't depend on a big job. It doesn't depend on a job at all, in fact.

I can't know where you are on your own journey presently, but I can assume that since you have picked up this book you must have reached a turning point in your life. Or one of your loved ones is anticipating that a turning point is headed your way. Retirement maybe. Or just a slowing down. Perhaps you are wondering what's next.

Or maybe you are searching for confirmation of your current resting place, or you are actively seeking suggestions for a new direction, perhaps a detour that sounds intriguing. Before we can securely make that decision to choose our next experience, I think it's helpful to take an inventory of where we are now; what we have learned that supports our life's purpose; where we think we could have done more; what disappointments we have grown accustomed to and forgiven ourselves for. Life isn't always pretty. Nor is it expected to be.

When I look back on my life, what experiences or accomplishments please me the most?

If I had to defend my choices above, what would my defense be?

What is it about those experiences that didn't "make the grade" that bothers me the most?

What was I doing when I was the happiest? Can I repeat that experience? If not exactly, in some form (e.g., raising children but now volunteering at a school)?

What did I struggle with earlier in life that wouldn't hinder me any longer? What has changed to make that so?

On my deathbed, I want to recount for my loved ones the many times I truly felt their love and what I hope they remember me for.

15

Roses Rather Than Thorns

We can complain because rose bushes have thorns, or rejoice because thorn bushes have roses.

—Abraham Lincoln

Actively, yet quietly, developing a peaceful perspective is the key, the one and only key I've discovered, to calm the running tapes in our mind, tapes that accelerate the chaos we feel within. Seeking to shift one's perspective away from the all too common turmoil, turmoil that generally isn't any concern of ours anyway, is a beginning. A beginning for a far more peaceful life, day by day, hour by hour.

Perhaps it seems that I am obsessively focused on living the peaceful life. Certainly many of these essays have peace and its attainment as the core message. No doubt there are other states of mind nearly as valuable as being at peace. However, I have yet to meet a mature man or woman who hasn't longed for greater spells of peace.

I think we are lucky, very lucky indeed, to be in charge of our state of mind, a state of mind that sees roses rather than thorns. Blaming someone else for our anger or hopelessness, or crediting them with our happiness or good fortune, means that our lives unfold entirely at the whim of someone else. I know I don't want to have my present or my future in someone else's control ever again. I lived that way quite willingly, yet at the time unknowingly, the first four decades of my life. That kind of life no longer calls to me, thank God. I'm not sure it ever really *called*, but once I surrendered my power to others, which was second nature to me, I was trapped nonetheless. And I crawled into that trap while still a child. For years I was trapped. Letting others have the responsibility for my actions, opinions, and feelings took me off the hook. Yet, because I turned my life, my emotions and actions, over to the "care" of others, I lived constantly on the edge of fear, never knowing where their choice or behavior would take me next. And I didn't know how to change my predicament.

But something did finally change. I still don't know what triggered it, but I did finally have a shift in perception. I finally saw what I was allowing to happen. Did this come about because I simply got tired of others' choices? Perhaps, but not necessarily. What I do know for certain now, and it's all I know for sure, is that I want to be in charge of my life from now on, which means stepping up to the plate and inviting God to help me select every action I take or opinion I favor. It may seem awfully late in the game to be making this choice now, but I adhere to the premise that it's never too late to start living a better life. And one of the keys to that better life is reclaiming a peaceful perspective. We were all born with one. And too often we bartered it away, decision by decision, when in the company of a stronger person. Let's stand tall and take charge. Peace begins with each one of us. If not now, when?

To be more peaceful, I plan to . . .

To spread peace wherever I go, I promise to . . .

To bring benefit to the world around me, I will . . .

16

Teachers of Perspective

Perhaps you haven't thought much about the role perspective has played in your life prior to reading these essays. But it's been a big one, I assure you, and over the years you have honed either a positive perspective or a negative one to near perfection. Whichever one we most often grab in the heat of the moment painstakingly paints the perspective we have about life. The good news is that we can more consciously choose to paint, thus project, a positive perspective, assuring that the "picture" that is us will be far different from what it was. Nothing stands in our way but our failure to make a different choice. In your life, who influences your perspective?

Let's pause a moment and think about the many people who show up on our path regularly. They are not showing up willy-nilly. Some are frequent visitors; quite possibly we envy a few of them because of their demeanor. Maybe they are easygoing, most commonly happy and willing to be helpful to others, all traits we admire. Many are family members, some of whom we look forward to seeing. Some not so much. The nosy neighbor drops in too. Don't ever discount her or dismiss him as unimportant to the development of your perspective, even though you may dread seeing them approach your door. You might be looking at one of your most important teachers whose every action or word is nurturing your willingness to be more accepting, a decision that shifts your perspective from negative to positive. This may be the very reason they are in your life.

On the other hand, maybe you are serving as their teacher, the one who can help them shift their negative perspective into one that is more genial. Demonstrating a new way of seeing may change everything that follows from this day forward in his or her life. No encounter is superfluous. That fact is worth rejoicing over. From the moment I embraced that idea, I was free of the dread I felt about every person who troubled me in the past, particularly those who had manhandled my perspective.

Because it's a worthy pursuit to make a list of our many teachers to date, list the primary ones in your journal, and acknowledge the specific gift that resulted from their presence on your path. And remember, not all gifts looked good when first received.

For example: Echo was one of my teachers. She was the first to introduce me to the concept of sacred contracts, an idea that was fortified by reading books by Caroline Myss. Initially I was frightened by the idea, but over time, this idea has completely freed me from the prison of guilt I felt over some of my past behavior. I know now that everything I did and everyone I met were agreed upon before I woke up in this world.

Now it's your turn to consider your teachers. The importance of this can't be overemphasized. Pick your primary teachers, regardless of how you evaluated them initially. What demonstrates they were teachers?

Now let's turn the tables and consider all those for whom you served as teacher. Don't underestimate your value to them. Your paths intersected quite by design. You had talent or knowledge or compassion that was very much needed by them at a particular time. They would not have appeared otherwise. If you are failing to think of anyone right away, take a timeout to meditate on your life and the many people you met.

Folks have not quit seeking you out, even though youth has passed you by. Who are they and what have you shared lately? The student/teacher exchange lasts a lifetime. A full lifetime.

Without a doubt, your life has been well lived. Some actions might have been improved upon. Some "students" handled with greater mastery and compassion. And your lessons were offered more than adequately. Often we still have one lingering thought about our past that haunts us. Feel free to share it here, for no eyes but your own. The very sharing of it is the best way to bid it goodbye.

17

Seeking Solitude

Seeking solitude as preparation for "changing our minds" opens the door to our future. Meditation is too little valued. "The more man meditates upon good thoughts, the better will be his world and the world at large," says Confucius. Without much effort, every one of us can have a positive impact on the world at large. It's as simple as choosing our thoughts with greater care. Every thought that we hover over becomes a bit more indelible, and when the thought that has taken center stage in our minds is an expression of love, we are affecting the universe in a good and peaceful way.

But not one of us is forever free from the occasional dark thought or dismissive demeanor; and when the inevitable happens (and it always does), our job is to quickly acknowledge what we are harboring in our minds and seek, *at once*, to shift our perception, to change our mind, in order to be better stewards of the universal mind. What a lofty job description.

I cherish this awareness in this last quarter of my life. Why? Because it means my life, my very existence, will never become superfluous to the constant hum of the world around me. Not one of us is without purpose, even when our contributions seem minimal to us. An expression of love, an act of kindness, a prayer for a friend or even a stranger, are the activities that change the world, making it more inhabitable moment by moment. And there isn't one among us who is incapable of offering one tiny gesture.

Before going one thought more, let's pause and consider what has transpired in our minds already since arising this morning. Let's consider each thought we have harbored so we can make whatever adjustment is necessary to ensure that we are impacting our world in a loving, healthy way.

Let's revisit our day so far.

What thought are you now uncomfortable with?

What thought do you wish you had coddled instead?

How different might your day be looking right now if you had been more protective of your thinking process?

How fortunate that what we thought only a moment ago holds no sway over us *at this moment,* unless we allow it to. This surely doesn't seem like a very profound realization, but it's one I didn't cotton to, and for sure never embraced, for the first four decades of my life. I so willingly gave my mind away, to whomever was nearby, sharing whatever opinion, pleasant or unpleasant, was being expressed. I was a chameleon. And I didn't even know it. Having a mind, a life of my own, was a foreign concept. I was sure that if my thoughts ran counter to yours, I'd soon be discarded for a more agreeable woman, a fear greater than the fear of death. Greater than the fear of *death.* What a powerful, lingering admission. And I didn't even recognize how little I thought of myself.

But now I do. Now you do too, or you wouldn't be interested in or comforted by this book. What thought are you trading in at this very moment? Perhaps a thought that served you very well last year but fits no longer. Let me share one of mine so that you get my meaning. In past years, I was prone to politely, but swiftly, letting others know when I didn't share their political or religious views. I wasn't bent on arguing, but I felt that if I said nothing when a companion shared his or her view, they might think I agreed with them. And if I didn't, I wanted them to know. I have gladly given up that idea. I may share where I am at, but more likely I'll let the moment pass. And it has empowered me, a realization I had not counted on. (There will be more on this topic in later essays.) Now it's your turn.

What thought or action can you let go of? And what can you replace it with?

Our personal power is hefty. Honoring it is both good for us and good for those who look to us as teachers.

Let's get back to meditation for a minute. That's where this essay began. In our quiet moments, we can fashion the person we want to be. With eyes closed, we can envision her holding forth with others, being who she has always longed to be. The power of this exercise cannot be overestimated. Who we see, we can be.

Who do you want to be now?

18

Take a Day Off

In this world it is not what you take up but what you give up that makes you rich.

—Henry Ward Beecher

What a foreign idea to most people. The ownership of stuff is how wealth is generally measured. The more one has, the richer one must be. But I sense a growing trend among some. It seems that baby boomers and seniors like me, and the generation just entering the workforce, value the less material: nature, the mind, spirituality, the family, play, solitude, *and even the choice to do nothing at all for a time.* This trend, though still limited in scope, is not invisible. Nor has it failed to make an impression. And for this I think we can breathe a sigh of relief. It's suggesting that we take a timeout. Everyone. Our worth is not in our stuff *or our accomplishments.*

What's the point of this book, then? you might be thinking. It's time-consuming to read. It was time-consuming to write. Obviously I'm not sitting on the sidelines resting in solitude. I'm held fast to my computer, day in and day out, exploring a wealth of ideas, some of which I share with you, the reader. But I take time away too. And I'm making a practice of extending those times. I want to practice that which I see being preached by the enlightened few. Enriching our lives with the nonmaterial is creating a space for new growth, new awareness, new habits. Unfortunately, old habits die hard. And I am very practiced at my old habits. Like many of you, no doubt.

The title of this book, *Living Long, Living Passionately*, is shorthand for the philosophy that has claimed my heart. Frankly, at seventy-five, I have rather easily accomplished the living long half of the title. And I do expect to live another decade. Maybe two, in fact. Living passionately has not been difficult either, while working. I love my work, whether writing, speaking, planning, or creating a program. However, I want to cultivate more passion around doing nothing. *Nothing at all.* And I'm not sure I can do that with ease. Time will tell. What I am doing here, now, is offering you suggestions that I need to also do, right along with you, the reader. I am making suggestions for how to experience the quieter, less intense life. The desire to slow down has surfaced many times in my life. I have been telling family and friends that I am going to retire. Someday soon. But the way to slow down, let alone retire, lacks clarity. But here goes . . .

———————————

To begin, let's greet the day expectantly, together. And then let's pause, long enough to invite the God of our understanding, whomever that might be, to have a say. I suggest that we sit in silence, with our eyes open or closed, for no less than ten minutes. During the time of silence, imagine God, or a guardian angel if that suits you more, conveying to you her hopes for us today. If nothing seems to come at first, let's be patient.

Now let's write for five minutes about whatever we are feeling. If you received a message, share that. If nothing came, that's okay too. But before abandoning this quiet time, let's thank our Higher Power for the love and protection we are offered daily, even when we are not aware of it.

Perhaps you aren't sure where I'm leading you in this essay. *I simply want you to slow down. I want to slow down too.*

Life doesn't need to be lived in the fast lane. Make a decision right now to do nothing all day. And if you can't commit to this because of an important engagement already on your calendar, take tomorrow off. Completely off.

This is my day off. I will catalogue in my journal all the ideas for things to do that I am willing to discard, for this one day only.

How do you feel taking charge of your life today, discarding all that you had previously felt you simply had to do? What images come to mind that illustrate this new freedom? Compose an affirmation that you can return to at any moment, on any day, when you realize you are about to do something you have no real passion for.

Feelings?

Images?

Affirmations?

_____

And before leaving this essay, I want you to thank yourself and your Higher Power for being willing to change directions. What you did, what I am also working to make a practice of, is to literally step aside, close the door, little by slowly, on the work I so lovingly do, day in and day out.

We are all the better for it. One and all.

Now take a long, slow breath and let the inner joy rise up. Thanks be to God.

19

Now We Can Really Live

Life will give you whatever experience is most helpful for the evolution of your consciousness. How do you know this . . . ? Because you are having it.

—Eckhart Tolle

Every one of our experiences is specific to us. Every single experience! Tolle knows this. So does the God of our understanding. The wisest philosophers throughout history would quickly agree too. What a profound idea. What a simple idea. And what a comforting idea when we *lean in to it.* It clearly means there is no reason to question any experience. Or to shrink from it. No reason to deny any experience either. Or doubt it. And certainly no reason to waste time categorizing our experiences as those we need versus those we don't. They all have made their visits as divinely orchestrated, at the right time, and in the company of the right teachers needed for each specific lesson. This is a statement you can take to the bank!

Are you currently happy? I surely hope so. Your past has delivered you to this point, *an encounter with me, as a matter of fact, through the pages of this book,* and it's my intent to help you squeeze understanding and joy from your past. I believe this will ready you for finding more joy in every lesson that lies just ahead.

And if you aren't happy right now, perhaps it's because you are feeling anxiety about the undetermined future. If you have forgotten that every person, every past experience, every past moment was "wearing" your name, you just might be wallowing in doubt about all future moments. Couple all of those feelings with entering your sixties or seventies, and you may be fretting that there is not much of the good life yet to live. But I say, *on the contrary*. Now we can really live. We are free from the uncertainties of the past.

Before getting bogged down in doubt, suspend any disbelief you might have about the necessity for each of your life experiences for a moment, and begin a list in your journal of a few significant experiences that have occurred in the last twenty or so years of your life. My point is for you to see how divinely orchestrated our experiences were and are, leading us from one to another, nary a coincidence among them.

After a list of ten or fifteen has come to mind, take each one and close your eyes, envisioning it as it was. In some, you will recall and relive the drama. In others, you may feel the angst or the sadness all over again. But purposefully they arrived, were absorbed, and then departed, readying us for whatever was to follow. Always readying us for the next encounter.

Surely, that format for our lives (i.e., the specificity of how events unfolded) won't change. But we can assume a more active role as co-creators of our future experiences, if that appeals to us. Let's dream.

How do you want your remaining years to look? What comes first to mind when you envision them?

How do you imagine a particular change might affect other people and ancillary experiences? What will your "picture" look like as it unfolds?

What would please you the most about the remaining decades of your life if you could manifest your most perfect picture of the future?

I want you to realize you have this power. You really do.

What's the first, next step on your agenda?

Rest in peace. Your heart's pure desire is headed your way.

_____

20

Writing Your Story

Understand that any expression (words, actions, etc.) that is not loving is a call for healing and help. Regardless of the form it takes. Respond to it with love. Always.

(A paraphrased principle from A Course in Miracles)

We can't change the world. (How we wish we could.) We can't change anyone in the world. (No matter how hard we try.) But we can change how we will respond in the world of others. And every time we choose to be loving or accepting or understanding or forgiving of any person or situation that initially disturbed us, we are adding great benefit to the universe. *The entire universe!* Does this seem unreasonable to you? Unfathomable? Or too lofty to be believable? If yes, think again. It is how the scales of life are balanced.

Close your eyes to the world for a minute right now so a memory or two of when you softened an encounter with someone else can bubble up. As soon as one comes, please write it down.

The importance of this suggestion is that it makes you and me fervently conscious of our impact on others. Each experience during which we respond with love is making our universe a kinder place for others to inhabit. It improves our condition too. Our actions, in this regard, are both selfish and altruistic. There's nothing negative about that. What we do for and to others, we are always doing for and to ourselves. And this means that when we are snippy or condescending or hateful or dismissive, we are treating ourselves in the same negative way. Any action reverberates right back to us, much like a boomerang. It makes good sense to express only love. Surely that's what we prefer experiencing too.

Now let's take a few moments to recall when we were less than loving. When we took issue with someone or reacted poorly in a situation. Close your eyes. Let it gently arise in your mind. Share what it was here. This is for your eyes only, so be specific.

If you could have a do-over, describe it. How does the do-over make you feel? Might you have amends to make?

———————————

Switching gears now . . .

Let's try our hand at story writing. Don't be afraid of the idea. No one among us is incapable of creativity. And this story is yours, *the one you want to live*. Close your eyes. While they are closed, imagine yourself in the company of someone, or many people, whom you care deeply about. You are preparing for an adventure you have always wanted to experience. It's yours to have right now. In this dream, you are living it. Live it to its end. And then open your eyes and write a description of it, of you in the experience, of someone else too. Include every detail you can recall. Make it sing with detail and reverberate with meaning.

This story you just wrote can be your next real-life experience if you want it. The operable question is: do you? I've heard it said, and I fervently believe it to be true, that whatever we imagine ourselves doing can become our reality. Further, I've heard it said that we'd never dream an impossible experience. It simply wouldn't enter our minds in any state of consciousness. If we can dream it, we can live it! We can make it happen.

Perhaps this reminds you of "vision boarding," an activity for manifesting our heart's pure desires. Many believe, wholeheartedly, that we can draw things to us if we "see" them first as already "captured." If you are experiencing some doubt about this, suspend your disbelief for now and move forward, as though you believe. Believe like a child believes in the tooth fairy.

But doing so means planning the first steps.

Write in your journal about what you need to put in motion first. What would be the next stage of the dream? Let's envision how the next stage of our life looks with this dream manifesting.

Not every reader will find success with this exercise, but it's one a person can return to whenever the mood strikes. Or boredom sets in. The point of this is simple: our lives depend on the choices we make, and our choices can be as far-fetched as we want. The only wrong choice, ever, is one that will harm others. We must be ever mindful that whatever we do, or dream of doing, will have consequences. Can we live with the consequences? But even more than that, can others live unharmed by our consequences? Never forget that every expression we or anyone else makes reflects love, or a call for healing and help. If your dream, your story, was in response to someone's call for healing and help, you are fulfilling the dream of the God of your understanding too. Meeting someone, anyone, where they are with an open heart is fulfilling the best story ever written.

If you are already living the best story ever written, then bravo! If not, decide to live a story that manifests your desires. As quickly as possible. It's the way to balance the scales of the universe.

———————————

21

Impacting Those around You

*Ask: What does this person [standing before me] need?
Instead of thinking about what you want, practice asking
what the other person needs. See how you can help.*

—Leo Babauta

Living passionately, as the book title suggests, can happen in
so many ways. It may involve travel, here in our country or
abroad, or going back to college. It may be resuming an earlier
craft such as painting or photography. Possibly volunteering at
a neighborhood school as a tutor or serving as a mentor for
some young person who needs a caring adult in their life. The
Boys & Girls Clubs of America usually has a list of youngsters
who need direction and someone to show an interest in them.

However, we can "stay in our own backyard," as the saying goes, and simply take notice of who is directly in front of
us on the path we have chosen for now. My point is that we
don't have to complicate the assignment. Look around you.
Whoever is present is on assignment too. And he or she needs
acknowledgment, before they need anything else. Perhaps they
will need nothing more than that, or they might need a lot
more. It's your opportunity, regardless, to help them find what
will make them whole.

Unfortunately, aging hasn't healed all the inner wounds of
the human community. For many, those wounds have been
exacerbated, in fact, by the myriad trials of aging. While it's
true that some people age ever so gracefully, others stumble

often and can't always get back up. And if we can, through nothing more than simple kindnesses, bring a smile to the face of a wounded soul, we will have demonstrated how passion looks in this instance.

To live long and passionately is not beyond the realm of possibility for anyone in America. In all of the western hemisphere, the odds are in our favor. We represent modern society and we have, at our fingertips, riches of many kinds. And since this is the case, I'd venture to say for everyone who has selected this book to read, the impact even a few thousand people can have on the communities we share is nearly beyond our imagination.

It's time to make a short list of the obvious ways we can impact those who stand before us. Here are three. You think of some more that specifically fit your lifestyle.

- Make a point of looking the first stranger you see (at the grocery, the taxi stand, or the doctor's office) in the eyes and nodding or saying hello.
- Engage at least one stranger in conversation.
- Invite a neighbor who doesn't get out much to go to lunch, a movie, or shopping when you go.

The point of this is that passion is a decision. And it's an attitude. We can feel inspired about anything at all. And every time we are inspired, we model for others greater possibilities for their life too. Inspiration has visited every person reading this sometime in this last year. Share what that was in your journal.

Before leaving this essay, is there something you feel you need from others? Asking for it doesn't guarantee we will get it, but no one knows we want it if we don't ask for it. To live passionately with a little help from our friends is good. Remember, we are allowing them the same opportunity others give us when we offer help. Giving and receiving are the gifts that complete the sacred circle of life.

What do you need? Who can you imagine seeking help from? What do you think their response will be?

People must give away what they have, to receive more of it. Let's each do our part. Now. Today.

———————————

22

Improve a Little

See everything. Overlook a great deal. Improve a little.

—Pope John Paul II

This quote by Pope John Paul II is delicious in so many respects. It's humble. Realistic. Manageable. It embodies a touch of humor. It contains all the elements of living well. Perhaps not perfectly, but well. And for these words to have come from Pope John Paul's lips makes them all the more interesting as admonitions. They represent the perfect philosophy for those of us who want to live meaningfully as well as simply. Be careful observers, he says, but don't live to be critical. And better yourself where you can, but go easy throughout your day.

I'm imagining a room full of parishioners hearing him speak those words, and on their faces smiles break out. Each knows how to improve a little. But most may not be in the habit of overlooking a great deal. If each of us could overlook even a few "deals," we'd help to make this a less contentious world.

Perhaps in our careers we were saddled with a lot of power because of the positions we held in our companies or organizations. Some of us managed that power (*i.e., we saw a lot and knew what to overlook*) in a way that freed others to do their best, to flourish. Others of us ran such a tight ship that creativity might have been stifled. That was then. This is now. And encouraging others to enjoy whatever they may choose to do, whether it's painting or bird-watching, golfing or playing bridge, tutoring or taking a class just for fun, and seeking that encouragement for ourselves too, is a wise and worthy way "to improve a little" while we help others to do likewise. Being cheerleaders for the human community is an activity in this stage of life.

Let's assume that you have the rest of this day, after reading this short essay, to do whatever would please you. What would that be? Make a telephone call to a friend you haven't seen for a while? Write a letter instead of just sending an email to a really special friend. Maybe it's trying your hand again at an old hobby, one that has been left untouched for a few months or years. Make a list in your journal of things that interest you. Include in the list some activities you have never tried before but considered doing a long time ago. Maybe include something that seems farfetched, even. Be daring!

Making a list such as this is meant to serve as an impetus for moving out of your current comfort zone. It's also representative of your heart's pure desire if you dig deep enough. You don't have to share this list with anyone else if you don't want others to know what you are up to. It's for your eyes only, but having a list has always helped me gain clarity about where I want to go next. What's most important about it is it reminds us that we are interesting people, still very alive and with good ideas, no matter what age we are. Getting old is a state of mind. Living youthfully and richly is a state of mind too. It comes back to choice. Everything comes back to choice. Pope John Paul suggests that we choose to live "lightly." I think that's a mighty fine suggestion.

23

Dream List

If you had no fear, what would you be doing today? Diane Conway, a woman I met about twenty years ago, wrote a book based on her interviews with people. Her primary question was, "What would you do if you had no fear?" The responses were amazing. What was even more amazing was the fact that some of those people formed a small support group to encourage each other to accomplish their dreams. The point of my mentioning this here is because I think we sell ourselves short. We get into a rut about our station in life and are too easily satisfied with standing still. We very seldom believe that dreaming is worthwhile and that our dreams are remotely attainable. They are just dreams, after all. Unfathomable dreams.

I'm of the opinion, after seventy-five years on this planet, that no dream visits us that can't be fulfilled. If it comes to us, we can do it! Maybe not instantly. Perhaps we need to complete some preliminary steps before we are ready to tackle the dream, but the idea itself wouldn't occur to us if we didn't have the capability to achieve it. For instance, perhaps your dream is to walk the Camino de Santiago. A friend of mine had this dream and she has now made the pilgrimage of five hundred miles three times, and she plans to walk a thousand miles next summer. Could she have done it when the idea first came to her? No. But she began to train. Over the next few months she walked daily, in all kinds of weather, until she could comfortably walk at least twenty-two miles a day. She took the necessary preliminary steps.

For her, the journey was spiritual. Perhaps that helped her be committed to the training. But my point is this, if we think it, we can do it. There must be something each one of us has tucked away, a dream that perhaps we have never dared share before. Here is the place to share it. Here is the place to gather your resources to pull it off.

I have dreamt for a time of practicing a craft of some kind. I tried watercolors three or four years ago, and while I enjoyed the process, I wasn't particularly good. Watercolors are not forgiving enough for my talents. But I haven't given up on the idea of painting. What I want to try now are acrylics or oils, or both. They are far more forgiving for the rank amateur. Even though I wasn't a great watercolorist, my husband did hang my three best paintings in our kitchen, and they look quite nice. I'm not ashamed of them at all. Putting a frame around *any* painting makes it look pretty good.

What is your dream? Maybe you have two or more, in fact. Don't be reticent. List them in your journal.

Chances are there are some steps you will have to take before going after your dream. I had to find a teacher. Then buy supplies. My biggest step was setting aside the time to do it. Each week before going to the painting class, I had to give myself a little pep talk. I doubted my skill. I certainly didn't think I had any real talent. I still don't think I am a talented painter. But my perseverance paid off. And perseverance is a worthy quality to strengthen, regardless of what we are persevering in. I persevere at golf at least once a week too. Am I good? No! Do I play anyway? Yes!

What are the steps you need to take to prepare for fulfilling your dream? Write a list.

How will attaining this dream change you? Might it lead to other dreams? What I learned from fulfilling mine is that I am rather crafty. I took up knitting next and got great satisfaction knitting baby blankets for an organization that helps young mothers. However, the most important thing I learned is that, should I choose to retire (and I actually plan to semi-retire at least), I do have many dreams that call to me. I won't be sitting with empty hours on my hands. Travel, arts and crafts, playing better bridge. And golf. Pursuing short story writing. Even though I have made my living writing and doing workshops for many years, what I haven't succeeded in is publishing fiction. That's on my dream list. At this very moment, I put it at the top of my dream list.

What's on yours? Remember, nothing is too outlandish or too unattainable. If you can imagine it, you can find the way to do it.

24

Doing More Than Nothing

In any moment of decision, the best thing you can do is the right thing, the next best thing is the wrong thing, and the worst thing you can do is nothing.

—Theodore Roosevelt

Theodore Roosevelt was our twenty-sixth president. He was a smart man, progressive in his political outlook, and he faced many adversities with great strength, as so many born leaders do. The above quote is intriguing because it suggests we can't simply duck our responsibilities. Doing nothing in whatever situation faces us is more than irresponsible; it's destroying the game plan of everyone on the periphery who was or is affected by the situation in question. We must step up to the plate and fulfill our roles when others are involved, or we bring to a halt a plan that was initiated by someone else before it reached us. Being a necessary contributor to a much bigger picture is exciting. It's also demanding, can even be unrelenting, and on occasion is thankless. We may still have a part to play even when no one cares, no one takes notice, or people downright dismiss our contributions. In fact, that's how it often plays itself out.

If we are suffering from the need to be acknowledged for our contributions (and who doesn't want the recognition at least occasionally?) when we reach retirement, it's almost a certainty that we will be disappointed again and again. If we do or did contribute primarily because of our need for praise, we are in for some pretty big letdowns. Let's take, for instance, volunteering to be part of a neighborhood council. They are often saddled with making decisions that affect many people, the majority of whom are actually strangers to one another, and then trying to enforce the rules that uphold the decisions. It sounds so simple when first agreed to. After all, the rules make sense! But then one person raises a fuss about a rule he doesn't like, and as the enforcer, you become the bad guy or gal. Suddenly you find yourself on the receiving end of nasty emails or phone calls, and what had begun as a volunteer duty has turned into a nightmare.

Our strengths while in the workforce can become liabilities during retirement. Others may want us to take charge of situations because we were successful managers before retirement. It may even be a feather in our cap to be called upon in this way, at least initially. But management with no real authority can be extremely time-consuming as well as stressful. Even worse, undermining. Trying to cajole people into adopting a new way of doing any task, after they had been doing it another way for a few years, even a few months, is like trying to take a favorite toy away from a child because he isn't sharing it. As a matter of fact, some adults behave far more poorly than children when confronted by changing rules.

The experiences that await us as we transition away from full-time employment to full or partial retirement are varied. Some folks have been saying for years what they were going to do when retired. At the top of the list for many people is travel. Adult education programs appeal to many men and women whom I have met. Becoming more skilled at bridge, golf, knitting, or any number of crafts, as mentioned in an earlier essay, is what satisfies the longing that some feel after they have closed the door on the profession that fulfilled them for so many years. If there is an emptiness, and it's normal to feel that void, it haunts us until it is filled.

I bring up this topic in multiple essays because it is the situation I will soon confront. Who am I if I am not writing? Who am I if I am not leading a group in a seminar? Who am I if I am not making a significant contribution to a conversation, to a casual gathering of friends, to a 12-step recovery group?

The question I need to lay to rest is this: Must I be "performing" in some fashion to be considered worthy? My hope is that it matters little, if at all, whether I do or say anything in any group I'm a part of. And I have an inkling that I am not the only bozo on the bus who thinks I need to be leading anything. My guess is that most people are far too self-absorbed to give much thought to what anyone else needs or doesn't need to do.

The crux of this situation, or any similar situation, is that a meaningful replacement for work that was extremely fulfilling is sought, and it's wise to have a few ideas for filling the long hours lined up to consider before closing that door for the final time at the office that has been a second home for so many years.

Making a list of activities that might hold my interest in a sustained way comes first to my mind. I say sustained because short-term activities are always plentiful. Making a dent in that pile of books next to the easy chair or on the nightstand, writing letters that are long overdue in response to queries received in the Christmas letters that get sent every year, antiquing that old table that's been in the basement for years now, or sorting through the (gasp!) hundreds of pictures that have filled more than a few boxes and bags over the decades—an activity that is mentioned on nearly everyone's to do list when they contemplate retirement. But most of us need a reward of some kind if we are to be genuinely committed to a particular activity. And how we define reward is very subjective.

An activity that would reward me is writing a piece of fiction that passes muster with a small publisher. Actually, I have been saying for some time that I want to explore self-publishing.

Maybe self-publishing is the best outlet for my fiction. Additionally, on my list would be a commitment to tutoring school-aged children. Once upon a time, I taught elementary school, and even though the curriculum has changed significantly (I retired from teaching in 1969), I'm sure I could boost the egos and the grade point averages of children who wanted to learn.

I know that everyone reading this has a dream tucked away of something you'd love to do. It really doesn't matter what it is. Simply having something that lights the fire within is the only requirement. If you honestly can't think of anything that calls to you, look in your local paper for volunteering opportunities. And pick one of them. Right now, pick one of them. Write it in your journal.

And go, tomorrow, before you second-guess yourself. Getting off the dime, as the old saying goes, sends you on your way. Life will begin to be just as exciting as it ever was before. And you won't look back. You won't. All the good stuff now lies ahead of you. Give yourself a week of this new stuff.

Then return to this essay and describe who you are now. In full and colorful detail.

I sure hope you are having as much fun as I am having steering you through this maze of new thoughts, new commitments, and new future evolutions.

25

Pay Attention to the Moment

It is a mistake to try to look too far ahead. The chain of destiny can only be grasped one link at a time.

—Winston Churchill

The outcome of every experience will be revealed to us at the perfect time, and not one minute earlier, regardless of our pleas to receive it yesterday. It will come in a perfect way, and from the people who needed to be part of the experience too. There are no accidents. Remember? The people we need to know will make their way to us. What we need to know will tap us on the shoulder. What we are to do with what comes to us will be spelled out, mostly by nudges, our inner feelings, or the spontaneous comments made by the people close at hand. No matter how unconscious we seem to be as we travel through life, we can't avoid or step around the business that we need to attend to. This has been true all the years of our lives. And it will remain true for all time.

I'm comforted by this information. I hate missing out on things. During our so-called productive years, most of what we needed to attend to was very apparent. And it came to us piecemeal. Most of us no longer need to be productive in the same way, but life still unfolds in a piecemeal way. And there is generally no hurry anymore. The life of deadlines is, thankfully, behind us. But no doubt we put deadlines on ourselves anyway. We deserve freedom. We can give it to ourselves. We can give it to one another too. The time for rejecting deadlines is now!

What should concern us now is this: *Are we feeling joy?* Are we looking forward to each moment as it heads in our direction? Let's be alert! It is the only moment there is. And after it has been experienced, another one will come. And then another. And then another.

Eckhart Tolle offers such beautiful detail about how life comes to us as a gift, moment by moment, in his book so aptly titled *The Power of Now*. There simply is no other moment but this one. And if we miss it, sidestep it for some reason, we are sacrificing life—not only our own life but the lives of others too. Each time one of us squeezes the life and joy from the moments that we are privileged to experience, we multiply the joy felt throughout the universe. What an awesome privilege. What an awesome gift.

As an exercise in paying attention, for the next twenty minutes, keep a log in your journal of every thought that passes through your mind: every exchange between you and someone else, every action or choice not to act that you make.

The point of this exercise is to make us conscious of how mindlessly and inattentively we live. Each moment is far too precious to be cast aside with so little consideration. There are no repeat performances for the moments of our lives. They come once, and then they go.

Giving ourselves the pleasure of spending whatever moments are remaining in our lives involved in the activities that bring us joy, and perhaps offer joy to others too, has no comparable alternative. Live wisely.

26

What to Do Today

You don't know what to do today? Listen to the travelers on your path. Listen to what's being said beneath their audible words. Look into their souls. See them deeply. They came to you quite by intention.

For many of us, we have come to the close of the day in our professional lives. However, we still feel vibrant and focused. Being sixty or seventy doesn't feel all that old. (And isn't, by the way! Take it from the seventy-five-year-old!) We know we aren't ready to turn out the light on life. But many of us are at a loss as to what we might do next.

The best place to begin exploring this big unknown is to start with a list of all the activities you were ever involved in. Perhaps as a youngster you loved a certain sport, one that isn't too dangerous for older, more brittle bones to undertake. Maybe you wrote poetry. Were you ever a volunteer at any time in your life? The time you have available to you now allows for giving back to a few select organizations. Any community of any size has needs galore. And they have hands galore too. Getting the two together takes little more than a phone call or two.

If you are still at a loss, simply enjoy the solitude of this new freedom. Perhaps you aren't meant to get involved with any activity right away. I'm inclined to believe that what or who needs my attention will wander my way eventually. I don't have to go seeking. I will be sought. You will be sought too. But if you are too impatient to wait on the seeker, simply make it a point to listen very carefully to every voice that speaks to you. One of them has a bigger message than you initially heard.

It's a bit like solving a mystery sometimes. We are pieces in a very large jigsaw puzzle. And not until enough pieces have been played, can we see the bigger picture. But in the meantime, the richness of life is quite apparent by the joy we experience in simply having brief, seemingly superficial encounters with the men and women who, like us, are just wandering around looking for connection. I think that's the magic word, in fact. Connection. We want the safety of being joined with others. Not abandoned just because we are no longer necessary to the profession that claimed so many years of our lives.

You will find your place now that you have made the choice to free up your life. It may take a few months of stalled beginnings, but the activity that will include the people who need to be within arms' reach of you will draw you to it. Like a magnet, you will be attracted to the people, the actions, the joys inherent in the activity. Every one of us has a very particular place we are meant to be. And we will get there, in time, to fulfill our purpose with the people who need us. Isn't this a most comforting idea? We are always at the right place at the right time with the people who are significant to our destiny. Always we meet one another. Always . . .

Now close your eyes. Let all extraneous thoughts, no matter how intriguing they seem to be, slip away. *Be still and allow yourself to hear the voice of your inner guide. He has been waiting to get your attention.* Now pretend, just for fun, that with your guide's help you can see what this right place is and who these right people are. Describe *in detail* all that you see and feel.

What's the most unexpected awareness about this picture you have drawn? Did a particular person show up in your picture show that took you completely by surprise? Can you imagine what your payoff is going to be? And can you guess what lesson you will be imparting to others?

Life consists of a series of joys, one following another, if that's the mindset we adopt. And for every one of us who adopts that attitude, an additional person someplace on this planet discovers joy too. Thank you for the contribution you are making.

———————————

27

Making Small Efforts to Improve the World

How wonderful it is that nobody need wait a single moment before starting to improve the world.

—Anne Frank

I have been utterly amazed on many occasions by reading a quote that is attributed to Anne Frank. How could one so young be so wise? Perhaps it is because she was destined to have a very short life, thus she had to share a full lifetime's worth of wisdom while still a babe. One can't help but lament the awful tragedy of her life, and the lives of seven million other Jews. And yet she offered us so much love and wisdom and forgiveness in those very few years. She was so much more than her age would have suggested. And for that we are blessed.

The above quote is so clearly about taking personal responsibility for the world we share with one another. She knew what it meant to be a victim of circumstances, but she also knew that she had an opportunity to live a responsible life, restricted though it was. Each one of us knows, too, what living responsibly means. But the circumstances of each responsible act will depend on where we are and who we are with. The decision simply needs to be made that no opportunity will be ignored.

However, there are actions we can always take that might serve as substitutions for specific responsible acts. For instance, passing on to someone else a loving thought can be substituted for a responsible act that might be calling to us. I think it's worth remembering that it's not always what we do that matters, but the way in which we do it. Are our actions kind and thoughtful? Do we overlook the small inconveniences others may cause us? Are we prepared to look the other way rather than make an issue about a situation that really matters very little?

I think it's a rather interesting idea to consider, for a moment, what small efforts we might make to improve this world. Many things come to mind, don't they? Easy things, in fact. Lending a hand to someone at the grocery store who seems to be a bit unsure of herself perhaps. Allowing the person walking across the street in front of our car some extra time is a very thoughtful and easy offering. I, for one, appreciate it when others do this for me. Not one of us is too busy to slow down and smile at the individuals we pass on the street, in the stores we frequent, or at stop signs while driving. We may think we are too busy to take the time to notice others, but, in fact, that's the only important "assignment" any one of us has throughout our lifetime. Regardless of age and status. *The only one.*

Take some time now to think of your typical day. Make a list in your journal of those things that would come naturally to do that would improve the world, ever so slightly. Just ever so slightly.

Now make a point to do these things during the course of your typical day.

There are two points to this exercise. One is to take notice of how you feel during and following the gracious acts you performed. My hope is that you will feel a sense of wellbeing for having shown a kindness to another. The second is getting a commitment from you to make this kind of thing a regular part of your day, every day. It takes little or no planning. Nothing more than willingness. The big question is how committed are you to making this world we share a better place?

To better instill this plan in your mind and your day, let me make a suggestion. I have found that it's beneficial to share with others the success of some change I am making in my life. Hearing the plan out loud has a way of focusing me. Perhaps it will work this way for you too. Before going any further, choose with whom you will share your plan.

Name him or her. Tell him or her.

What kind of inner shift have you experienced since trying these exercises? Describe it in as detailed a way as possible.

I'm guessing there was an inner shift. There always is when we honestly devote our attention to trying something new that brings benefit to others. In fact, I have discovered that my own life is exponentially enhanced whenever I do something good or kind with no expectation of a response. It's a bit like the movie *Pay It Forward,* a very touching story with Kevin Spacey playing a school teacher who interests a particular young boy in the idea of anonymously doing something kind for some unsuspecting individual. The end result is a very changed boy, a changed teacher, a changed mother, and a changed community. The good deed idea reaches its tentacles far, showing that when someone does something good for us, we feel inspired to do likewise and pay a kindness forward into someone else's life.

It takes so little, really, to make this a better world. A gentle nod to this person, holding a door for that one. Making the decision, every day, to do even one thing that lessens the load for someone else is my challenge to you. And I guarantee you will feel lifted by the experience, and you will begin selling others on the idea too. This is a mighty fine legacy to leave in your wake.

If you feel like sharing more about your experiences with this, do so here.

———————————

28

Fulfilling Your Potential

The most common commodity in this country is unrealized potential.

—Calvin Coolidge

Perhaps you have never considered, before reading this quote, that you have unrealized potential. After all, many of us have arrived at the final quarter of our lives. Aren't we done yet? Haven't we *spent* ourselves? The fortunate answer is no. We aren't done until the final breath is taken. *We aren't done until we have completed the life we were sent here to live.*

Perhaps you haven't thought about your life in terms such as these. Being *sent here* carries a far different meaning from simply being born. I had not seriously considered that we were born specifically for certain assignments until reading the books of Caroline Myss, the spiritual intuitive I have referred to many times in this book. To refresh your memory, she says in *Sacred Contracts* that we make a contract, an agreement of sorts, on the "other side" with each soul we will encounter after being born into this life. This means, of course, *that not one of our relationships is accidental.* Each one has been preplanned for the lesson we both agreed to experience.

When I was first introduced to this idea early in my forties by a friend who insisted that she knew it to be true, I doubted it. But then after coming upon the idea again when I read Myss's book, I felt instant, comforting relief. Like so many of us, I had experienced myriad encounters throughout my life that had troubled me, some gravely, others only slightly. However, I felt a quiet joy when I learned that each one of them, regardless of their content, was a learning lesson. And I was both teacher and pupil, switching roles as the lesson dictated.

I am not suggesting here that you need to share this belief, but I do want you to consider the ease with which you can look at your past with a different understanding now. In fact, what I suggest we do in this essay is reconsider some of our past experiences in light of this possibly new awareness. If Caroline Myss's name is new to you, google her when time permits, but for now, let's explore the past together. The lessons you've learned have been many, quite fruitful, and *always intentional*.

Who is the first person you remember, from your childhood, who didn't seem easy to be with? Perhaps she or he laughed at you or declined to be friends when you so desperately needed one? If childhood doesn't bring someone to mind, how about your teen years? Take a few moments here and now to quietly close your eyes and remember once again the experience, the feelings, the resolution, if there was one.

When I was young . . .

What's the nagging realization you have about these memories that rushed back to you?

Do you feel peaceful about the awareness? If not, why not?

What I'm driving at here is that there is so much more to our existence than a superficial overview would suggest. Our experiences are rich with meaning. Every one of them! Not one of them should be overlooked or dismissed as mere entertainment for the ego. Each experience has contributed to the wholeness of who you are now in this latter stage of life. We have truly deserved each and every experience. I don't mean that to sound harsh or insensitive if some of your past has been painful. I just want to emphasize that we couldn't be where we are now without each past experience. No doubt there were a handful of them that you hated. That's no doubt true for everyone reading this. Me too. But let's revisit a couple of those and look at them with fresh, wiser eyes. Can you see how they made you a better person? I'll share one of mine, and then I want you to do likewise.

When I was a young girl, before I had hit my teens, I was sexually assaulted. It happened more than once by the same individual. He was a shirttail relative and I was far too timid to pull away, resist, or tell anyone. I simply let it happen and was troubled by it for more than thirty years. When I finally talked it over with a cleric, he suggested I work with a therapist. The therapist suggested I write about it. I did. The details of all that happened aren't as important as the ultimate result. I eventually had an experience with forgiveness that was profound. And that experience had an impact on every other experience in my life. I see the entire scenario as a very necessary part of my journey, and I can fully accept it as a sacred contract, just like Caroline Myss explains in her book.

Now it's your turn. Recall at least one experience that you can comfortably see now as a blessing even though at the time of initially experiencing it, you were troubled.

I remember . . .

I hope you are becoming aware of the necessity of each thread every experience has contributed to the tapestry that is your life. What beautiful tapestries we have woven. Being grateful for the pleasant as well as the less-than-pleasant occurrences that make up our past is what prepares us for the host of experiences that are awaiting their time as our lives continue to unfold.

Before leaving this essay, take some time to remember all that you have to be grateful for. Make the list in your journal. Share the list. Then thank your God as you understand him.

All is well. All is always well.

———————————

29

Who Will You Bring to the Party?

Ask how you'd live your life differently if you knew you were going to die soon, then ask yourself who those people you admire are and why you admire them, and then ask yourself what was the most fun time in your life. The answers to these questions, when seen, heard, and felt, provide us with an open doorway into our mission, our destiny, our purpose.

—Thom Hartmann

Looking back over our lives no doubt gives many of us reason to pause and think, *Why didn't I do that when I had the chance?* Fortunately, there is still time to fulfill some of our dreams. Dreams, particularly waking dreams, often indicate what we'd like to do. And yet how often we push these dreams aside, sure that we are needed to take care of far more important activities. Think again!

Taking to heart what Hartmann says in the above quote, if you were soon to die, you very well might choose to follow the dream, *so why not follow it anyway?* Not one of us knows just when we will take our last breath, so living out our dreams feels like a great idea. Doesn't it?

What have you not done that you'd always hoped to do? Take a particular trip, perhaps? Make contact with someone you knew very long ago? Take a class in a subject area that always interested you but felt too disconnected from the profession you had settled on? The time is now. Make a plan. No matter what it is, there is no time like the present for making this adjustment to your life.

I am going to . . .

How does it feel to make this promise to yourself?

Now let's follow Hartmann's second idea. Who are the people you have admired and why did you admire them?

This is important because those we admire can become our role models. It's never too late in life to select a new role model.

How will your behavior change? Take a moment now to meditate about the way you will now show up in the lives of others. After envisioning the "new you," create a scenario that reflects it.

How do you feel now? Are you appreciative of the fact that we can change who we are at any age?

And last but not least, when did you have the most fun in your life? What were you doing? Who with? Why did you stop doing it? How would it feel to start doing it again?

There is no time like now to give it a try. Perhaps it has to be scaled down somewhat. For instance, maybe you were playing bridge four nights a week, and you no longer drive at night. You can still play in the afternoon. Or maybe you entertained friends for dinner every weekend, and now that feels too overwhelming. You can still entertain, but maybe have potluck meals or order in from a deli. Or better yet, invite folks to come in the afternoon for dessert only. It's generally the socializing that appeals to us anyway, isn't it?

The point, of course, is to be willing to adjust our expectations. That's really all that has to change. Life, at any age, is as rich as we make it. It's who we bring to the party that matters, isn't it?

As a last exercise here, who do you envision taking to your next party?

_____

30

Make Yourself Smile

Putting a smile on someone's face before they fall asleep is all I hope to do. If I can do that, I will feel like I have been successful.

—Jimmy Fallon (paraphrased)

I am a fan of Jimmy Fallon, and since he has taken over *The Tonight Show*, my husband and I have been recording the show so we can watch it at an earlier time the following night. Fallon has sent me to bed wearing a smile more than once. My purpose for highlighting this in a book of essays on living long and passionately, is because this philosophy fits so well with the goal of this book. Is there any other more worthy gift any of us can give one another than what Fallon hopes to give? I think not.

This small book of essays can't change your life in any way without your consent, of course. And why should you want to make a change? Perhaps you don't. But then again, I'm thinking that since you selected this book, you must be on a search for something. More peace, perhaps? Or joy. Or the possibility of wearing a smile more often. Maybe you are simply acknowledging to yourself, as I have done, that you have entered the last quarter of life. How many years remain isn't mine or yours to decide, but what is ours to decide is how we will spend those years and who we will be in those remaining years.

For starters, I know that I want many experiences that continue to make me smile. I hope that the essays I write for you in this book give you some reasons to smile, or at least feel inspired to seek joy in the activities you undertake. Smiling is a decision we can make. And this very moment is as good as any moment to make it. Smile at the letter carrier, the clerk at the grocery, at the driver of the car next to you at the stoplight. To smile is the quickest way to ease the tension we so often carry in our muscles, tension that has so often been initiated by our desire to control someone else's actions. Of course, we can't control anything about anyone else. No matter how justified we think our demands are, we are out of luck if we think we are in charge of anyone but ourselves. Period.

How lucky we are that we aren't in control. That fact, in and of itself, should make us smile. Many reading this have already had reason to celebrate this, but whenever we learn it is the right time for us. As I've said in other essays, there are no accidents! Who we meet, where we meet them, making friends of strangers in the process, and where we are going next have all been determined. We will unravel the rest of this glorious mystery called life incrementally, and in the company of the right people and at the right time. This realization can put a smile on our faces right now. We need not fret. Ever again. We can relax and let go. We aren't in charge; God is. Whew! This is something to smile about!

Life is so much less complicated than most of us have made it over the years. Because I want you to really appreciate this, let's take a moment to look back.

Can you recall some past situations that seemed monumental and beyond resolution that got resolved quite smoothly without your help? Name one or two. Describe how the resolution occurred.

Do you see that you didn't have the power to resolve the situation?

That's how life works when we stay out of the way. It's not that we are bystanders to our lives, *but we can't expect to* feel like wearing a smile very often if being in charge of the actions of others is the work we think we are here to do. We will simply fail, repeatedly, if we make what others do our life's work.

Many of us have now completed the formal phase of our work life. But most of us still seek activities that motivate us, experiences that are meaningful and rich in rewarding ways. We aren't looking for the same kind of return on our investment of time, but we want to know that what we are doing counts in some important way. Don't we?

There are many choices we can make, but we have to do some soul searching and also be willing to "try on" a few activities before we settle on the one or two that really fit us. Perhaps these questions will help you zero in on who you are now, in this next phase of life:

Do you like working alone or with others?

Do you want to work with a particular age group, say as a tutor for young people? Or perhaps with older adults?

Why is this your choice?

Do you want feedback on what you are doing?

If you do, how will you handle the negative feedback, if there is some?

Do you want an activity that schedules you for a specific time?

Do you want variety in the assignment?

As you envision it, what's your dream volunteer work?

And remember, if you can dream it, you can have it!

All of these questions will help you zero in on the kind of work you might select. It's your happiness at stake. Remember, it's you who wants to go to bed smiling, and just maybe helping others to go to bed smiling too.

31

Changing Ourselves to Change the World

> *Everyone thinks of changing the world, but no one thinks of changing himself.*
>
> —Leo Tolstoy

This philosophy is espoused by many. I'm sure Tolstoy wasn't the first to voice it, and current great thinkers won't be the last. It's a very simple idea, actually, and one that I personally love. I think it has a way of right-sizing us. We lament how awful the world is all too often. Radio and television bombard us continually. "How can people, blah, blah, blah?" we whine to one another. A simple, yet very productive, question we might pose instead is, "How can I see this differently?" If we dare to ask that question, we will note immediately how changed the world will look to us. Changed completely, in fact. And how refreshing this new perception is.

Only by changing ourselves can we hope to bring about change in the world around us. Wishing the world would change carries no wallop. Changing our minds about the world, on the other hand, is powerful beyond belief. What's exciting for me as a writer, and hopefully what you feel some excitement about as a reader, is the inner power we can instill in one another to make this a better world for all of us to inhabit. I'm not talking about monumental changes. I'm talking about the tiny changes that don't go unnoticed. We can offer these up as many times every day as we want.

I read many years ago that Mother Teresa was supposed to have said, "Be kind to everyone, and start with the person standing next to you." Can you imagine the impact for change if only a handful of people on every block in every community practiced it, just once every day? The ripple effect would transform the country. And as happens with the hundredth monkey effect, the change would eventually cross oceans, circling the globe, and nothing would be the same. Anywhere.

As we contemplate how to spend our remaining years, whether traveling, volunteering at a local food shelter, pursuing a new vocation, tutoring or mentoring those individuals who need a special hand to find their place in the world, or filing the hundreds of photos that have accumulated over a lifetime, we can, concurrently, bestow kindness on everyone we encounter. This tiny action, blended in with whatever else we choose to do, will change us at the same time that it changes those around us.

It may seem that our remaining years need to be focused on something far grander than carrying the message of kindness. Let me assure you, there are no limits to what our choices might be. We are only limited by the mind that shies away from risks. All that's being suggested is that along with the chosen activity, regardless of what it is, coat it over with kindness.

I'm personally struck nearly every evening by the closing story on NBC national news. The anchor generally shares a heartwarming story of how someone has changed the lives of a group in need by a simple act that grew, attracting the interest of many, and the result was many lives being transformed by selfless acts of kindness. I know that every time I listen to one of these stories, I'm nearly moved to tears. So very little needs to be given to a very few for so much to actually change. Being a part of a change that really matters is a challenge everyone reading this could make a commitment to.

Let me help you make a plan that you can carry out. Even if you haven't made a choice yet, let's pretend in order to get started.

Let's assume you have settled on an activity that excites you. What is it?

Let's assume further that you have begun interacting with those people who are also involved. How are you feeling within when you quietly retreat for a few moments to reflect on the people and the activity?

Share your thoughts in your journal or with a close friend.

Making a gratitude list is a familiar way to get in touch with all the goodness in our lives. Perhaps you have had reason to do this in the past. I well know the impact it has had on me, and when I'm in a difficult place, the quickest way to get out of it is to begin making a list, right then and there. When I am in an ungrateful state of mind, it impacts every thought I have and all the actions I take. The words I share too. Being grateful for even the smallest of blessings is the daily reminder most of us could be changed by, and it's so simple.

If you haven't ever made a gratitude list, or at least haven't made one for a while, there is no time like the present to claim the gift we receive from making a gratitude list.

I'll start one too. I am grateful for the good health I enjoy at seventy-five. The wonderful partner in my husband Joe. And I'm expressly grateful for the gift of writing. It is the central core of my existence, along with the workshops and seminars I facilitate. Every man and woman whose eyes meet mine are gifts to me, straight from God.

Now it's your turn. Name a few things you are grateful for.

The point of this exercise, in case you have forgotten, is to shift our perception away from the negative places we go, often so unconsciously, and into the mood that makes us want to offer a hand or a word of kindness to the stranger who has been quite explicitly sent our way. Our opportunity with this stranger is the change the world is waiting for. Let's recall Tolstoy's words: we can't change the world, we can only change ourselves and then see how the world will be changed.

Our power is hefty. Let's always use it to benefit others.

32

Reaching Out

Every day do something that will inch you closer to a better tomorrow.

—Doug Firebaugh

I love this simple suggestion. Don't you? It's not asking for anything really big. It's not asking for anything beyond the capabilities of anyone reading this essay. Inching closer to a better tomorrow can be the result of hundreds of simple activities. For instance, being careful to treat everyone we meet today with respect insures that we will awake free from guilt tomorrow. Offering to lend a helping hand to someone in trouble is a sure-fire guarantee that we will feel necessary to the journey we are sharing with others. Saying a simple hello to the people we pass on the street, or greeting a cashier in the grocery store, or occasionally taking a special treat to a neighbor are all examples of acts that will create a better tomorrow for us and those we *purposefully* live among.

The list is endless, actually. Writing a note to a friend or even sending an email or making a phone call that has been long overdue are often overlooked though easy and ideal ways of inching us closer to a better tomorrow. However, I do want to make the point that our focus shouldn't necessarily always be on seeking a "better tomorrow," *but on living a better day today.* And every time we reach out to someone else in a loving, attentive way, we are fostering for them a better moment, and we will enjoy a better moment too.

Let's consider some of the better moments we have experienced and offered to others during the past few weeks. It may take some quiet contemplation to recall, but quiet contemplation is always good for the soul.

Make your list in your journal. It's not quantity that matters but quality of those kind acts. And remember that every kind act honored you too.

What pleases you most about having made a difference in the lives of these other people?

What additional signs of love and respect can you imagine now that you have begun this undertaking?

Following a simple suggestion such as this is life-changing. Even more, it's culture changing. One small act by each one of us can change the world for every one of us. I think it's worth the effort. Do you?

Would you consider being so bold as to ask friends and family members to join you in this effort? Perhaps making a list of the first ten people you would approach will move this idea forward in your mind.

And last, but surely not least, would you consider asking them to do the same?

I thank you on behalf of the community of souls that we share.

33

Influences

Few things affect any one of us more positively than being both the receiver and the giver of heartfelt and frequent acts of kindness. The shift we each feel as the result of someone else's kindness inspires us to "pass it on." When we do, the miracle begins and then repeats itself over and over and over again as first one and then another passes on an intentional act of kindness. We change just as much as those around us change. We are buoyed up by the attention we both give and receive. It's an amazing experience, in all honesty. Certainly one we should all take advantage of.

We have all been impacted by the lives of others, particularly those men and women who have inspired us in some important way. In this essay, I'm asking you to quietly reflect for twenty to thirty minutes, and then:

Name ten of those individuals.

Tell the circumstances of how you met each one.

What were the details of their influence?

Next tell exactly how knowing them has changed you over the years. It's quite possible that the longer ago the meeting was, the more influential you now realize they were.

Allow plenty of time for this activity. There is no hurry. This activity will reveal some very important information. You may well discern why you chose the work you did for much of your life. You may also see quite clearly the kind of friend you try to be. Your chosen mate may also be a reflection of one or more persons you met along the way. Perhaps you see now that some of your traits are the direct result of meeting specific people.

Now take some time to fully absorb what you have learned through this activity. Address each of the following suggestions:

Name the ten people in the order of their influence on you.

Choose the three most important influences.

Which lesson are you the most grateful to have learned?

Take any one of these influences and create a timeline showing how that specific influence played out; that is, when and with who.

Switching gears now:

Name ten people you think you have influenced and in what way.

Whom do you wish you had spent more time mentoring while they were in your life?

What pleases you most about your interactions with the younger generation?

Is there someone you think you failed along the way? How would you make it up to them if you could?

Pat yourself on the back for a job well done in answering these questions.

And last but definitely not least, before moving on to another essay, attempt to contact the individuals who influenced you along the way, by note, phone, or email. Tell them what knowing them meant to you. Thank them for their input in your life. Express to them, if you can, a few of the specific results of what you learned from them. Honoring others in this way is the finest gift we can offer.

34

We Become What We Think

Our life is shaped by our mind; we become what we think.

—Buddha

I'm sure this quote by Buddha isn't an unfamiliar idea. Perhaps you didn't attribute it to him, but undoubtedly you have heard an idea similar to this uttered many times over your life. It's a popular notion among psychologists and psychiatrists. Gurus of the self-help movement have relied on it for years as an explanation for why people behave as they do. It's also considered the easiest way for people to change aspects of their behavior. *"As we think, so we are."*

A book I wrote a few years ago, *Change Your Mind and Your Life Will Follow*, offered a dozen simple principles for changing ourselves by changing how we think. It's important to admit that we aren't stuck in a pattern of behavior unless we choose to be. That's the fortunate news. It was always our truth, in fact, even though we may not have embraced it or allowed it to influence who we were or who we were capable of becoming. However, even though we are in the latter stages of our life, there is no reason not to change something about ourselves, even now, if we fail to be at peace with our choices, our friendships, our anticipations about how the future looks. That's very good news, indeed. It is never too late to *create* a happy life.

I personally consider this a blessing. Hopefully you do too. There is no reason to let life slip by, assuming that we have no power to change that which we experience. That's the only thing we have the power to change, in fact, and it's not because we can change others. *Never can we change others. But we can change how we experience others.* Each and every other. That's because we can change our perspectives on everything and everyone. We sit, at any age, in the seat of power when it comes to observing and interacting with the world around us. How we do it is our choice, always. The childhood lament of "he made me do it" has been over for decades.

You may be feeling some doubt about this. We don't always recognize just how much personal power we have. Therefore, let's try an experiment. Surely there is at least one thing in your life you would like to change. I can certainly think of a few. For instance, I want to quit making snap judgments. I've been guilty of this trait my whole life, at times being better at not judging than at other times. But any judgment I/we make doubles back on us. What can we do to break this pattern? Here is what works for me. When I meet someone new or am in the company of someone who gets under my skin, I try to remember to pause. I say *try* because I know how easy it is to slip off the plan. But I have learned that what I see in someone else that I so quickly judge is a part of my personality too. Generally, it's a part of my personality that I hate, in fact. Pausing gives me time to rethink what I'm thinking.

Feeling unfairly treated is a trait that hounded me for years, particularly in my youth. However, falling back into that destructive self-definition is all too easy, even in these latter stages of life. Using the "pause button" on this trait is very effective too. For me, then, the practice of pausing is powerful. We each need a simple tool we can grab on to. You can use mine if you'd like, but for now, just contemplate what it is that you want to change. If it helps to close your eyes and look over the past couple of weeks of your life, do so. No doubt, that which you need to change will leap forward in your mind.

In your journal, write about the things that you want to change.

Along with pausing in the midst of thinking or making a negative judgment, as a way to prevent an unfortunate action, you can recall a fond memory about this person or someone else. A fond memory of anything or anyone changes the heart. Either or both tools changes who we are and what we are bringing into the universe.

Now can you reframe your response to life's challenges? How will your reactions and actions look?

For this day, I will . . .

I do hope you feel excited about taking your power back in the myriad situations that so easily rob us of being our better selves. What we bring to the universe is ours, and ours alone. Each one of us has a unique part to play, a unique gift to give. If we observe ourselves carefully, we will be able to discern that which we are and that which we are becoming. Some may think that in the latter stages of life, it's no longer important to work on ourselves. But your purpose isn't yet fulfilled if you are reading this. There is still time . . .

35

Listening for Messages

You cannot do a kindness too soon, for you will never know how soon it will be too late.

—Ralph Waldo Emerson

Most likely everyone reading this essay is, like me, growing older and slower, but feeling far from done in this life. I have been on the planet writing books and facilitating workshops for nearly half of my seventy-five years. And I've loved every minute of it. Those first few years and books were written while sitting in my big brown recliner holding pen to paper, and then the Apple computer became my tool, and it's where I have been for nearly twenty-five years, nurturing my love of writing. All of this has been coupled with our intense connection, yours and mine, in churches, classrooms, and auditoriums all over the world. I don't really want to bring to an end that which I love so much, but I know the time has come to make some changes.

Change. It comes. We resist. We even refuse perhaps. Initially. And then we remember, no change runs counter to the divine journey that is ours to experience. Then we absorb it. Sometimes we love it. Sometimes we continue to fight it. Regardless, it comes and that's where I am on this cloudy, cool spring day. I've lived long enough, steeped deeply enough in a spiritual process, to know that no change greets me unprepared. And yet, I find myself a bit unsteady at this juncture, not unlike the crossroads many of you have faced; and like you, no doubt, I am listening for guidance about this next phase of life, guidance that may come in the words of a song on the radio that gets my attention or a passage in a book that falls open at my feet. Or the half-spoken sentence that trails off from a complete stranger. If I listen, truly listen, my path will become clear. Of this I am certain.

I have surrounded myself with thoughtful friends and spiritual gatherings for decades. From one of my sources, I will get the inkling I need. For now I am simply moving gently through the hours and days and weeks of living, offering kindnesses wherever I can. I am convinced it's those kindnesses that open the doors to the messages that are wending their way toward me. Toward you too. I'm so happy that I read many years ago that Mother Teresa, when asked what might change the world, said, "Be kind to everyone and start with the person standing next to you." That pleases me. That comforts me. Nothing more do I need do this very day.

It may seem to some of you that this is a very simplistic way to chart a future, and that I need to dig deep and do specific research about the possibilities I might undertake in the days and years ahead. For many that is the way to go. For me, not so much. I want a less complicated path. I have always lived a less complicated life. My journey to who I have become, to this place where I now sit, with these many books under my belt and the many thousands of people I have met and interacted with over the years, developed organically. It all unfolded in an untethered way. With little or no direction. From me. I was never overtly in charge of the journey. I wrote because I yearned to know God. I felt most connected when allowing That Voice, Those Words to move through me. And then I spoke because I was invited. For no other reason did I speak.

We all got where we ended up because we listened to one suggestion or another. I intend to keep listening. And just today I heard a friend say she looked forward to my slower life, a life that would allow more time with her, playing bridge perhaps, or simply revisiting the stories we have experienced over the years.

I've done quite enough, actually. No doubt you have too. But the continuing desire to make a difference doesn't die for most of us. Choosing in what way we might make that difference calls to us. And in the meantime, shower your friends as well as your foes or the strangers in your midst with kindness. Simple kindness. And let the message that's been readied for you be delivered. It is on the way.

As I've said numerous times before, it's not what we do or what we did that matters. It's how open our heart was whenever we were in the presence of others. We can commit to that now regardless of how we fared in that respect earlier in life. What's in the past is gone. And doesn't matter. What's present now is all that matters and in this moment our messages are wending their way to us.

What do you hope your message is?

If I had my way, I'd hear . . .

And then I'd be excited to . . .

My life would feel more complete if . . .

And I'll come to understand that nothing matters except how I show up and what I do in that moment. It will look like this . . .

The next chapter of my life is being formatted now. Here is how I imagine it will look . . .

My blessings are so many. Let me share them . . .

36

Being in Charge of Who We Are

A person can make himself happy, or miserable, regard-less of what is actually happening "outside," just by chang-ing the contents of consciousness.

—Mihaly Csikszentmihalyi

What a powerful truth the above statement is. It puts me in mind of a book I wrote a few short years ago: *Change Your Mind and Your Life Will Follow.* We are fortunate, indeed, that our happiness as well as our misery depends on nothing and no one outside ourselves. Blaming others (spouses, bosses, kids, nosy neighbors) or situations (bad weather, heavy traffic, barking dogs, a job loss) for however we felt became a habit for some of us, a long-standing habit. It may still linger as a habit, in fact, but the empowerment that comes with knowing that no one, no matter how powerful they pretend to be or that we allow them to be, can make us feel bad or sad or angry without our full consent isn't easily squelched once experienced.

Being in charge of who we are in every instance, and how we feel regardless of the circumstances facing us, might be described as a natural high by some. Living above the fray feels safe. Knowing that we determine our own perspective allows us to move through the rigors as well as the highlights of any day with a much greater sense of purpose, wellbeing, and ease. We are not simply flapping willy-nilly in the wind. We never were. Nor will we ever be in the days and years ahead.

In all honesty, we have never been at the mercy of others. Even when we wanted to pretend we were, the truth was that we had willingly succumbed to whatever state of mind we were protecting. Was there a reason for it? Probably fear played a part on occasion. Perhaps it was simply the easy way out to shirk responsibility. At other times, casting blame for our circumstance simply felt good. We mistakenly thought if we made others responsible for the many ills of our life, we'd look better. If it weren't for them . . . and on and on.

Now that we are in what might be the last quarter of our lives, making every minute count for something is certainly appealing. It feels mandatory, in fact. At least from my perspective. I've had a great life. I really have. I've traveled the world, both for work and for pleasure. I've met tens of thousands of people who were seekers, just like me. Imparting to them the wisdom I have so fortunately acquired over the years, with the help of every person I encountered, was a gift. How I ended up in this position as a writer and teacher constantly baffles me, but I have felt directed by God every step of the way, once I had put the bottle down. And even before I had poured that last drink, God was in the wings. I just didn't know it, and would not have appreciated it or acknowledged it.

Whatever you were doing before you decided to pick up this book also had the hand of God in it I think. You may not share that assumption, and that matters not, but it eases my journey to believe that I wasn't the director of my journey, even though I had to agree to the terms of the trip. What matters to me now is that you and I have come face-to-face through the pages of this book, and that's not coincidental. Not at all. We agreed to the terms of this meeting a long time ago. Caroline Myss, a spiritual intuitive, would say that our encounter was agreed to even before our births.

Cast doubt aside for now, if you have some, and simply consider all that you had experienced in the decades before meeting up with me. Can you see a pattern emerging within the places and the people who crossed your path? There was one. Always there was one, and there will continue to be one. Our experiences are never accidental. Every one of them has applied an additional layer of substance, the substance that makes each one of us unique. And necessary to the whole of humankind.

———————————

Let's take some time to enumerate those experiences that were instrumental in defining us. If I go back to my childhood, I would have to say that writing stories and plays as a youngster grounded me in the awareness that writing could serve me well. Could comfort me. It allowed me to get out of myself. It allowed me to learn how to listen to an inner voice I didn't even know was there.

What is the first experience that comes to your mind that connects, even loosely, with the career that claimed your time for much of your life?

As I look back on that childhood activity, I'm thrilled with the awareness that the groundwork for who I was to become was being laid out, unbeknownst to me. It gives me a sense of wellbeing, even now, that what was true then will remain true, always.

Now cast another glance back over an earlier period of life. Many experiences will come to mind, no doubt, but choose the one that is gnawing right now. Maybe it was with a childhood friend or a first lover.

What stands out for you now in that recollection?

What was the experience?

Did it leave you feeling safe? Good? Fearful? Curious?

What thread from that experience has been woven into the fabric of your life currently? There is one. I assure you.

Now let's recall some of the happiest times in your past and the people who seemed always to be present when you were most happy. Close your eyes and take a few minutes to let these memories wash over you.

What was it about the people that so impressed you?

Can you see the part you played in the experience you savor now?

The point, of course, is to realize without a doubt that our happiness was under our control. It will be under our control in this last phase of our life too. In order to make the most of this last stretch, perhaps we can cull from those favorite experiences in our past a few that stand out and reclaim aspects of them, retool them, so to speak, for the benefit of who we are now and who we are on the verge of becoming.

37

Remembering Those Who Made a Mark on Our Lives

I recently heard someone suggest that we need to let those people from our past who significantly touched us know how much they mattered to our journey. Perhaps it was David Brooks, a columnist from the *New York Times,* who said it. It's in keeping with the kind of thoughts he shares both in his column and on the *PBS NewsHour* on Friday evenings. Regardless of who said it, it's vastly important. Honoring others by telling them our lives were made better by their presence is worth the time it takes to recall who they are and then track them down when possible.

I think the best way to approach this assignment is to look at our lives in decades. It's possible we won't come up with someone for every decade. Or perhaps some decades will produce more than a few names. The point is to both acknowledge that others did help us on our journey and then to give them the kudos they deserve.

Everyone likes knowing that they are appreciated. I get emails and snail mail from people all over the world who feel that my words in one book or another made a difference in how they are living their lives today. Every single time someone contacts me, it takes my breath away. I know that I am merely a channel for the God of my understanding. My words are simply what I hear as I sit at the computer. When they ring true to a reader, it's really God who has reached them. I'm so grateful for the part I played as the purveyor of the message. And I'm so grateful that the readers went to the trouble of contacting me. Each time it happens I feel like something very sacred has transpired between us.

Suggesting that you do this exercise isn't fair unless I do it too. So here goes:

When I recall the early years of my life, those years before college in fact, besides my parents who tried to guide my choices, even though I mostly ignored them, I was under the tutelage of Don Rivers, my supervisor at Loeb's Department Store in Lafayette, Indiana. I worked in the sportswear department from age fifteen (lied and claimed to be sixteen) until I was in my third year at Purdue. Mr. Rivers believed in me. He strongly suggested I go into merchandizing in college. I didn't follow his advice, but he did hold me to high standards, and I knew working hard and not waiting to be told what to do would pay off. It did. Every time he could give me a boost in salary or give me a new challenge at work, he did. I felt valued. It was the first meaningful job I had. I learned to work hard and to make sure he knew he could count on me, both qualities that served me throughout my life.

The last job I held at which I worked for someone else, those qualities I had honed in my teens actually got me promoted to the top of the heap. I became the boss of a twenty-five-million-dollar operation. Thank you Mr. Rivers, wherever you are.

Is there someone in your life who comes to your mind now? Even if you can't track him down, it will be good for your heart to think of him or her, write a note that gets sent or not. It's about the change within you that's also of value here. Remembering those who helped us along the way is also one of the many ways we shower positive ions into the atmosphere, ions that take us one thought closer to the tipping point that shifts the universe into a more loving experience for all.

I remember:

There is a break of a few years in my life before another obvious cheerleader comes to mind. I had a principal in the elementary school where I taught in St. Paul, who saw something in me I surely had never seen. His name was Ray Firnstahl. He considered me a master teacher. He convinced me I had a special gift with children, in fact. And I loved every minute I spent with them. I excelled, as did the children, because of his vision. That's the way it is with visionaries. They move all of us to do more than we had imagined we were capable of. Thank you, Ray wherever you are. Even though I left the field of elementary education, what I learned about the magic of encouragement from you has served many of my associates well, particularly those individuals who have looked to me for help over the years.

Who do you next remember? No matter how little you valued their input at the time, if they come to mind now, they mattered. Remember them in your journal.

The next individuals who pass through my memory are some of the professors who were instrumental in my pursuit of a PhD. I wasn't a scholar. I did work hard. But I also loved school, much to my amazement. I had been a party girl as an undergraduate. I really didn't give up the partying, but I took to graduate school like a fish to water. And writing was my forte. Unlike most of my colleagues, I never dreaded writing a paper. I relished every one of them. I was born to be a writer. I just hadn't fully realized it before.

And yet, had it not been for Chester Anderson, Mulford Sibley, David Noble, Mary Turpie, and Roger Buffalohead, I might not have mastered the mechanics of a PhD. Each one of them, in their own way, pulled me forward. They praised me, they gave me the freedom to pursue my specific interests, they believed in me, giving me the courage to believe in myself. To each of them I say thank you. I truly wouldn't be where I am today without you.

Now it's your turn. Who comes next to your mind?

I do hope you can see the value of this exercise. Remembering others and being remembered closes the sacred circle that includes us all. Doing our part to make another person know she mattered might well be the very gift that makes her life feel complete. Don't you want to be a part of that?

_____

38

The Greatest Gifts We Can Offer One Another

My life, by choice, is now more focused on the simple pleasures than was the case while in my fifties and sixties. Perhaps that's normal maturity. The body gets tired. The mind seeks freedom from worry. And with age, our relationships generally become less intense; if we are lucky, they mellow out. The expenditure of time, to make them more peaceful, has already been spent. Once we reach our seventh decade, we can breathe more deeply, I believe, allowing situations to be what they are rather than how we think they must be.

My guess is that you share these same thoughts. Or you are trying to, at least. But I believe it's worth our time, as we walk through the pages of this book together, to ruminate about a few of those greatest gifts. I have certainly learned over the years the value of repetition coupled with the practice of specific virtues. We might not be in total agreement with what these virtues are, but yours will no doubt be similar to mine. Let's begin with mine. You can add your own wherever it suits you.

The virtue, or gift, that comes first to my mind is *the gift of prayer*. When I was a youngster, my prayers were simple. "Now I Lay Me Down to Sleep" was the only one I knew by heart. Not having been raised in a very actively Christian home, praying before meals or at bedtime was not a big deal. Uncle George, when he was in a sober spell, offered up long, rambling prayers before our large family gatherings, but the meal wasn't held up if he wasn't to be found. However, prayer has become a mainstay for me. It quiets my mind and heart. I can do it silently, while with others, and I can do it ritualistically before meditation. I don't pray for things. I used to, of course. "Don't let Steve dump me, God." "Please let me pass this exam."

But even when the prayers were childish and pleading, they effectively helped me stop worrying. It reminds me of the proverbial God Box that every person in 12-step recovery is introduced to. The relief I got every time I needed to talk to God about a situation was palpable. I'd write down my concern, put it carefully in my God Box, and quite miraculously forget it. It worked because I believed it worked. My God Box was always full. The power of prayer can't be overestimated.

Even though I seldom put a prayer in my God Box now (I do still have it), I do have long chats with God on a daily basis. I put many friends and family members on my prayer list too. It relieves me of my obsession to worry about others when I "hand them over." When I hand anything over, I feel free.

Give some consideration, now, to the role of prayer in your life.

Do you pray regularly?

Does it offer you relief?

If you aren't in the custom of praying (and that's perfectly okay), how do you handle your concerns about others?

If you do pray, what's the primary benefit you have received from prayer?

Let's move on to another gift or virtue. I have many in mind for us to consider. The one that comes rushing into my mind next is this: *the gift of silence.* I grew up in a noisy family. My dad was often angry, so it wasn't unusual to hear loud voices and lots of cursing. I dreaded his coming home from work many days. You could tell by the time he got out of the car if supper time was going to be peaceful or loud. It never seemed to be simply fun.

I, too, became a loud, angry person. I fought him, tried to stand up for my mom and brother, and mostly suffered an upset stomach for my efforts. I didn't begin to appreciate the power and the effectiveness of silence until I made a commitment to the program of Al-Anon, and even though I have been active in that 12-step program for a long time, mastering the practice of silence relies on daily adherence. But I haven't explained why I think silence has so much to offer.

What is it about silence that makes it a virtue? I have thought about this long and hard and have written around this topic before. What I have to say isn't new. But that doesn't detract from the wisdom of it. Choosing to be silent rather than being engaged in a discussion that is headed into a power struggle pays off. I know. I have spent countless hours practicing this, sometimes successfully, sometimes not so successfully. Choosing to be silent, as long as it's not a resentful choice, is beneficial for a number of reasons.

First and foremost, it's a great demonstration to others that not every argument has to be joined. It's also an example of choosing peace rather than the alternative. I heard a great acronym at an AA meeting a few years ago. It was WAIT. It stands for "Why Am I Talking?" I'm certainly guilty of talking something to death. And I've been privy to others who do it too. Opting to be quiet, even once in a while, is freeing. It's like opening a window and letting the stuffiness out. If it's not a general practice of yours, consider making it one. Even for a week. It can add unexpected pleasure to your encounters with others.

Being quiet is an intriguing idea. Begin the practice of it now. Where it might lead you could be interesting.

What did you notice first when you made the choice to be quiet? Were others surprised that you didn't have an opinion?

How did it feel to say nothing?

Will you practice silence on a regular basis?

Why or why not?

The point of focusing on these simple gifts is so we realize we don't have to change very much to make our lives richer, easier, and of greater benefit to others. The next gift or virtue we can practice is offering rapt attention to the people who skate across our lives. It became apparent to me a number of years ago that there is no greater gift that we can offer another person than to be attentive to them. Everyone wants a witness to his life. Everyone deserves a witness too. We absolutely need to know that we matter. In this moment. In this relationship. In this family.

Being attentive to the people we encounter is the primary assignment each one of us has each and every day. This isn't the first time I have mentioned this idea, though in a different context, in this book. But its importance can't be overstated. Being the difference in someone's life, the difference that encourages them to do more than they had ever planned to do, benefits the universe. No matter how far-fetched that may sound, it's true. That which is expressed here, in this moment, with this person, makes its impact there in a matter of time. We are a part of the wave that moves the human race forward because of the attention we so willingly give. Or withhold.

Do you remember someone that paid you attention earlier in your life? What was the impact?

Do you feel prepared to repay that attention to someone else now?

Give some time, now, to choosing who you want to help make their mark.

The final gift I want to discuss in this essay is the payoff from shifting one's perception. Through the spiritual program, *A Course in Miracles*, I was introduced to the idea that we truly can see any situation we choose or any person we encounter differently, if we sincerely ask for help to do so. The phrase (it has almost become a mantra) I use is, "Help me see this differently." I am not beseeching God, necessarily, for help. I am simply opening myself up to the universe and quite willingly letting my ego go in that moment. This tool, or gift, has never failed me. I'm not sure how it works; only that it does. Surrendering to the universe changes everything.

Perhaps you would like to try it. I can't make guarantees, of course, but I do believe that your own life will change, just as mine did. I'm personally convinced that being at greater peace, which is the end result, is what we deserve in every phase of life, but particularly in this last phase. You will experience it. I promise.

And now for practice. Say to yourself:

When I am faced with a situation I'm uncomfortable with, I will seek to see it differently.

Practice this at least six times and keep track of the results.

It's time to move on. After incorporating a number of the ideas that have been offered to you in these first thirty-eight essays, some new ideas perhaps, some not so new, you may well be feeling that this last phase of your life will be the best yet. Frankly, that's how I am feeling. Moving into decade seven took my breath away five years ago. Now it feels great. It feels productive in a new way. But most of all, I feel empowered to take what I love doing to a whole new level. I hope you are getting to that place too.

39

It's Time for a Change of Pace

Let's look back over our lives and recall some peak experiences. It may take some time to sort out the memories. Because of my very checkered past as the result of my alcoholism and drug addiction, I managed to destroy more than a few peak experiences in the early decades of my life. Unfortunately, I destroyed what began as potentially good memories for others too. But there were some peak experiences that predated my drinking and many that followed my willingness to get clean and sober nearly forty years ago. It's to those I'll turn. I suggest you begin a list too.

I mentioned in an earlier essay that I was an author of stories and plays as a young girl. My friend, Bonnie, and I built a small, cardboard stage, complete with a curtain, furniture, and a stationary dog. We made puppets too, to tell the stories we had written. Was it her idea or mine? I no longer recall how it transpired, but we were proud. We got praised by all the teachers and the principal. Of course the kids loved the plays. They got out of their regular classrooms and came to a small basement room, the same room we used for physical education when it was raining outside. Bonnie and I hid behind a table covered with a blanket. The stage sat on top of the table. On our knees we manipulated the puppets and spoke the dialogue and loved the laughter from the kids.

I never guessed I would look at this as a peak experience one day, but indeed, I think it helped to propel me into becoming the "performer" I am today. Making others laugh at the stories I share in my workshops tickles me. It's the same feeling of well-being that I was introduced to sixty-five years ago!

I think the value of looking at the high points in our past is at least twofold. First, acknowledging that there were some high points simply feels good. Reliving good memories is another way of wrapping ourselves in a cozy comforter. And second, it points to an activity that we might choose to repeat, albeit in a slightly different way, perhaps. I know that for the rest of my life I will probably share, on occasion, some of the ideas I've written about in my books. Interacting with others makes me feel alive. And necessary. And absolutely connected. That's where my healing lies. That's where all healing lies, I believe.

Now it's your turn. Share one of your early peak experiences in your journal and toy with how you might revisit it, revamp it, so to speak, in this latter stage of life. I think that any memory of consequence is ripe for repeating. The format may change. The substance, not so much.

I remember . . .

Repeating it now might look like this . . .

Many of my friends have claimed peak experiences around their careers, schooling in preparation for those careers, or perhaps around motherhood or fatherhood. I can only imagine how giving birth to a first child might rank as one of the most cherished of all experiences. I didn't give birth, but walking across the stage to claim the honor of PhD ranked right up there for me. It was an achievement I had never imagined attaining.

Even when I began my American Studies master's degree program, I didn't plan to pursue a PhD. I did it simply because I had made no other plan for the rest of my life, and the man of my dreams hadn't invited me to join him for his relocation. With no defined future at hand, I simply moved forward.

Walking across that stage as a sober woman with my family in the audience marked my turning a page in my life. I was writing a new chapter. I didn't have any idea how the chapter would end, I just knew I could accomplish that which, heretofore, I had assumed was beyond me. And, indeed, deciding that writing was my forte, a requirement in every course I had taken, led me to authoring a host of books now numbering twenty-nine. And still counting . . .

Was there an achievement in your life that you look to now as a stunning turn of events? What was it and how did that experience inform your life? Might it continue to move you forward?

If you are like me, and you no doubt are at least in some respects or this book wouldn't have garnered your attention, you have had a plethora of peak experiences. Some of them with family members. Others with friends and colleagues. I think some of the most intriguing are those powerful experiences that happened with complete strangers. I had one a few years ago at the AA International Convention in Toronto. We rode a train every day between where we were staying and the convention site.

As is common in a gathering of recovering alcoholics, everyone is a friend. Saying hello and making introductions is commonplace. I was with a few friends, walking from the train into the center, making small talk with the folks around us. It's customary to say your first name and where you are from. Walking next to this woman, I said, "Hi, my name is Karen. I'm from Minnesota." She looked at me, and much to my surprise, asked, "Are you Karen Casey?" I said yes and she screamed. Loudly. "I can't believe it," she said. "I prayed, just this morning, that I would meet you here."

We laughed. My friends laughed. And I was once again reminded that my life is none of my business. It never has been my business, and it never will be my business. I was called to do what I have done. It was an assignment that I was more than willing to fulfill. I honed my love of writing in graduate school, and there was a purpose for it. A purpose divined by the God of my understanding. Indeed, meeting Kathy S. on that walk to the convention site was an experience I will always cherish. Who could have guessed that a lost soul like me would leave a mark on the world of recovery?

What is another of your absolute best memories? Now that I'm culling my mind for my own, I am inundated with them. Perhaps we should extend this essay. You find one and see how it has fit into the puzzle of your life.

Share it in your journal.

Because I am flooded with peak memories, let me share another one. I sat across from Mr. G, the final professor who had yet to approve my dissertation. The three-hundred-page document had been in his hands for more than two months with nary a response. The other four professors on my committee had glowingly approved it within a few weeks of receiving it from me. Mr. G was the holdout. I finally managed to get an appointment with him to discuss it.

He didn't actually look me in the eyes when he said, "This has to be completely rewritten." I gasped. After catching my breath I said, "But my orals are in three weeks."

"Not my fault," he replied. At that moment, a quietness filled my mind and I heard myself asking, "Would you be willing to go through it with me so I can understand your objections?" Much to my surprise, he said yes.

For the next three hours I heard nothing, really. But he was talking and I was responding. At the end of that time, he looked over his granny glasses at me and said, "I am satisfied. I'll see you at the oral." Both confused and relieved, I walked out of his office, searched for the closest pay phone, and called my husband. "The most amazing thing just happened," I said. "God came to my rescue."

I knew, without a shadow of a doubt, that my willingness to fully let go, to surrender in a way I had never before surrendered, allowed the God of my understanding to do for me what I couldn't have done for myself. This was, for sure, the peak experience that rose to the top of my list of memorable experiences. It's possible nothing will ever supersede it because of the certainty it provided me that I did have a Higher Power who truly had my back. I have never doubted, since that day, that I will always get the help I need if I seek it.

You have had many peak experiences, I know. I suggest you make a list of them here. Discern the impact these experiences have had throughout your life. They mattered. A great deal. Reviewing them will help you be aware of new ones as they are happening.

Looking back on your life, what's the most important experience you have ever had?

What's the most important thing you have learned?

Who's the most important person you have ever encountered?

What do you wish you could repeat before it's too late?

40

Stepping Aside

Yesterday I was clever, so I wanted to change the world.
Today I am wiser, so I am changing myself.

—Rumi

The drive to change "out there" so that we feel better "in here" is seductively powerful, some say addicting, and it is almost always disappointing. Getting someone else, anyone else in fact, to do exactly what we want them to do generally loses its luster shortly after they have done it. I used to be troubled by this realization, particularly when I had a lot riding on the change I hoped that they were going to make. So why didn't I feel satisfied and truly gratified when my plan was implemented? Why did the result that I had gerrymandered fail to sustain me? Hmmm.

What seventy-five years of living, coupled with forty years on a spiritual path, have taught me is that any action others engage in that feeds my ego, my desire to control, eventually leads to conflict and isolation. And I don't want to be separate from others anymore. I have experienced, on this spiritual journey, the joy of union, of communion, of sharing a moment in time with someone else that pleases us both. These moments, though intermittent, are referred to as holy instants. In this, my last quarter of life, I want to savor these holy moments. I want to create more of them, actually.

I have spent years practicing the behaviors that guarantee me moments of peace. There is no shortcut avenue to this quiet destination. However, I do believe peace is available to all of us. It won't elude us if we want it more than we want to control anyone other than ourselves. Let's think about this idea of control in greater depth. I know it's been my primary lesson in this life. It created problems in my first marriage. It continues to pinch me in my second marriage. I stub my toe on control many times every day. But at least now, perhaps because of maturity, I am willing to step aside rather than always insisting that I am right. Regardless of the circumstance. What a freeing feeling. Like Rumi said in the quote at the beginning of this essay, changing myself is far easier and wiser than trying to change the unchangeable.

Wisdom comes with willingness to shift our perception, I think. In our youth, the idea of giving in to how someone else sees a situation is anathema. One of the payoffs of aging, at least for me, is experiencing the joy, the relief, the quiet peace that comes with saying, "You might be right."

I'm guessing that the main thrust of this essay rings a bell with you too. We begin to think more alike as we age (as long as we leave religion and politics out of it, that is). But even in those arenas, sidestepping conflict is more appealing than when I was younger. What I want to bring your attention to now, however, are those ways in which you see yourself more willing to change.

———————

List a few situations in your everyday life in which you might be able to step aside.

My failed attempts to change others . . .

Primary ways I expect my life to change or feel as a result of my stepping aside.

The realization that the universe (the "out there") reflects our state of mind and our behavior lays on us an awesome responsibility. One that doesn't suffer fools. And yet, how lucky we are to be on the pitcher's mound for the game of life we are playing with seven billion other people. How lucky, indeed. I think it's wise, at this point, to recall some of those times when we played our part well.

What effortlessly comes to my mind are the many books I felt called to write over nearly thirty-five years. I know that the words my computer spelled out were dictated by a Greater Source than my own mind. And if the hundreds of responses I have received from readers over the years can be trusted, and I think they can, those readers, those members of the universe, have been positively influenced. For many of them, significant changes occurred. My part, my responsibility, was simply that I listened to the quiet, inner voice, wrote what I heard, and followed his directions. The rest is history, as the saying goes.

Now it's your turn. You, like me, have had an impact on the people assigned to you on your journey. There is no way to deny or ignore this. It's a fact of life. And your assignment with each person who came to you was quite specific, though it probably didn't seem so in those moments. Moving your minds back in time will clear the way for the past actions and thoughts to resurface, to be remembered.

What are some of those thoughts and behaviors that are claiming your attention now? They need to be acknowledged. And celebrated. The universe needed every one of them.

Before moving on to the next essay, let's simply pause and give ourselves a pat on the back. What we are doing, here and now, is a gift to ourselves. It's also a gift to those who are closest to us. We will see, very quickly, where we might have done a better job with that select group. Fortunately, life is still being lived. By them and us. And how we choose to behave in the many tomorrows that we will share is available for us to chart in a manner that will make us proud and them valued.

Let's try this small exercise, for starters. In this new day, I will . . . .

_____

41

Be Kind

Be kind whenever possible . . . It is always possible.

—Dalai Lama

This statement by the Dalai Lama reminds me of Mother Teresa's suggestion to "be kind to everyone and start with the person standing next to you." Both of them have served as great examples of how to make this world we share better for everyone. Interestingly, they both seem to agree that it's not about making grand, sweeping gestures in the circles we covet. It's never been about that, I'd guess. Rather, it's about showing up small, offering simple gestures that pay love forward. And love can be represented by a smile, a willingness to listen when a witness is needed, a shared moment of laughter when appropriate, or maybe a ride when a person's car isn't available. There's a multitude of gestures just waiting to be selected. Thinking up some new ones is even better.

Now that you and I have more time to devote to making these small, kind gestures, let's show our willingness to do so, every day perhaps, or at least once a week. For some of you reading this, it might even be your first step on this terrain. Or perhaps you have been making kind gestures for years throughout your life even, but doing it more consciously now is what I'm suggesting. Why? It's my observation that far too few people take the time to sincerely notice the many others who travel the same paths that they travel day in and day out. Mindlessly, we move through our lives. But it need not be that way.

Being present to and acknowledging the men and women who are within earshot as we move through the day is one obvious act every one of us can begin practicing *immediately*. And being noticed is an indication that you have mattered, a very important gift in this day, when too many of us are moving too fast, thus we notice too few. Let's stop. Now. And look around. Who do you see? Have you considered smiling at whoever is close by?

There isn't any complex preparation necessary for making this change in our behavior. But here are some simple suggestions for easing us in to the mindset.

—————

Consider these initial suggestions as meditative:

1. Go slowly.
2. Go quietly.
3. Form an intention about your plan. (Write it down.)
4. Carry it out. If you have more than one, take action on all.
5. Keep track of your actions.
6. How many were simple smiles?
7. How many were investments of time?
8. How many offered a quick payback?
9. Were any gestures ignored? Can you guess why?
10. What surprised you the most about this activity?

—————

The entire thrust of this essay is getting you to look around, getting you to notice the companions who have joined you on your journey. As I've said repeatedly, they have not haphazardly shown up. You selected them as your teachers. Likewise, they selected you. But to learn that which you came here to learn, you have to notice one another. You have to be present to one another. You have to truly listen to one another. Hopefully, in the process you have been kind to one another, too. However, those who are closest to us are often the ones we treat the poorest. Fortunately, there is time to make restitution. Let's make the plan to do so, here and now.

———————

Who are the people I want to show up differently for?

What actions am I prepared to take immediately?

What outcomes do I anticipate?

What pleases me the most about making this change in my behavior?

I will be committed to fulfilling this contract from this day forward.

Now sign and date this plan in your journal.

———————

42

Remembering the Little Things

Enjoy the little things, for one day you may look back and realize they were the big things.

—Robert Brault

For a change of pace, let's look back now. Let's look back and make a list of the many experiences that continue to stand out in our minds, experiences that seemed big and significant, along with those that were minor. List them all, since they have been recalled. The simple fact that we remember them makes them worthy of further consideration.

I'm thrilled to be looking back with you. I have a laundry list of memories, some pleasant and some not so pleasant. For our purposes here, I'm not going to draw a distinction between the two. They all contributed equally to the person I have become. If I could list them all, I would, but those that bubbled up first got selected. Here goes.

Some Memories:

1. I remember, as though it were yesterday, suffering nausea and intense anxiety while sitting in Miss White's second grade class as she walked down the aisle toward me. In her hand was the proverbial pencil that she used to repeatedly poke the top of my head. What could I have done to anger her? I never knew. I begged to be moved to another teacher. Neither my parents nor the principal would hear of it. Most Sundays were spent lying on the davenport, sick with dread that I had to go to school the following morning.

2. I remember my first drink, whiskey and coke, quickly gulped at the age of thirteen while no one was watching. It was a wedding reception and the attention, fortunately, was not on me. The warmth I felt throughout my body as the liquor slid down my throat was palpable. The memory of it now, sixty-two years later, is still palpable. I was certain it could heal the inner wounds that gnawed at me. But alas, I painfully learned that that was not to be the case.

3. I remember my eighteenth birthday and the carton of red Pall Malls that my oldest sister, Jo Ann, gave me as a gift. That was my rite of passage into adulthood. My father had asked each of us kids not to smoke before we were eighteen. His gift was a wrist watch, any one we wanted from the jewelry catalog. Of course I had already smoked, but I selected a watch anyway.

4. I also remember buying myself a necklace for that same birthday, telling my family it was from my boyfriend so they wouldn't think poorly of him for not buying me a gift. My parents didn't like him, and I didn't want the absence of a gift from him to add to their dislike.

5. I remember speech class in high school, and the joy I felt from giving prepared speeches in front of the class. I was selected to compete at the state level for our school but backed out at the last minute, not out of fear but because I didn't trust my boyfriend while I was out of town. It greatly disappointed my teacher. Of course I didn't tell her the real truth for dropping out.

6. I remember my boyfriend, Fred, in college. He was a terrific dancer. That was the glue that drew us together. He never seemed interested in kissing me. I found out some years later that he was gay. My dad said that he had always suspected that. It had never crossed my mind.

7. I remember meeting my first husband. I was drawn to him because he was smart, cute, loved to drink,

and had a red Buick convertible. We married for all the wrong reasons. Alcoholism and infidelity tore us apart.

8. I remember coming to believe that a Higher Power existed and had been my constant companion. And protector. My Higher Power had sent an angel named Pat to help me when suicide was imminent. Her knock at the door interrupted my plan, and she assured me that I was on the precipice of a significant spiritual breakthrough. I believed her, or I wouldn't be writing this book today.

9. I remember sitting across from one of the professors who was on my dissertation committee. He had just told me my three-hundred-page document had to be completely rewritten. I was stunned. The other four members of the committee had glowingly approved it. He agreed to go through it with me. I didn't hear his questions. Nor did I hear my replies. However, three and a half hours later he gave me a glowing report. God had spoken for me. This I know.

10. I remember sitting in my big, brown recliner having daily chats with God early in recovery. Those experiences became the written meditations that in turn became *Each Day a New Beginning*. I had never planned on them being a book. They were simply my daily security blankets. But the rest is history.

11. I remember the first workshop I offered. It filled a need in me. It continued to fill a need for more than twenty years. Now, at seventy-five, more time for quiet contemplation is needed.

12. I remember riding in my friend's car and announcing to her that I was going to retire at seventy-five. Now that I'm there, I know a full retirement isn't what I want. Just a slowing down.

Now it's your turn. Let what comes to mind first be the starting point. What's so very true is that you and I are a composite of every memory, good and bad. Each one left its indelible mark on who you are today. Every experience was necessary, or you wouldn't be reading this today. And you are exactly where you need to be. *Without a doubt!*

Be daring. Dig deep. Personal reflection can be a spiritual journey. Enjoy the trip.

43

Having Goals

The process of working toward a goal, participating in a valued and challenging activity, is as important to well-being as its attainment.

—Sonja Lynbomirsky

Some of you may think that placing your sights on goals is of little interest now that you are moving into this latter phase of life. And it's absolutely okay to be done, if that's your preference. However, I continue to hear from many people who believe that having a goal, having a reason to put on socks in the morning, is still extremely important to them.

Many who share this opinion are friends, but the greater number of them are actually strangers who have contacted me through my website or as participants in the workshops I offer. For these folks, the desire to seek fulfillment through some activity continues to call to them. And I say bravo. I say bravo to those who want to be done, more or less, and to those who still want to be busy, to move forward.

There is room for all of us. There is a need for all of us to fulfill that which continues to call to us. And the desire any one of us has to keep producing or working or volunteering is sacred—not to be ignored, not even to be taken lightly. It's part of the sacred journey we agreed to complete before we arrived here.

Like many of you, no doubt, I have been goal-oriented my whole life. It started in grade school. I wanted good grades, so I worked hard. Getting perfect scores in spelling and on math assignments was a big deal to me. And I wanted to read more books than any other pupil in class. Biographies were my favorite genre. I couldn't get enough of them. They fed my active imagination. They inspired the short stories and plays I so loved writing.

Goals kept school interesting to me. My success at attaining them prompted my desire to have a job, a job that paid me, as soon as possible. I got my first job selling tickets on kiddie rides at our city park when I was twelve years old. Having my own money to spend how I chose was intoxicating. And I never looked back. From that age forward, I always had a job. Always. Jobs gave me a sense of importance, a sense of completion, of belonging. I wish jobs had also filled the emptiness I so often felt inside. But that was not to be.

Nevertheless, I have no regrets about the hard work. I never even considered that a person could make the choice not to work hard. I had been raised to think of work as character building, an activity that insured my worthiness. Although my mother had not worked outside of the home until my younger brother and I were in junior high school, she amazingly went to night school, learned to type and do bookkeeping, and got a job for the very first time. That set an example that impressed me.

Not only was I amazed at her courage to go to school as an adult (she was in classes with students far younger than she was), but her drive to prove herself became eminently apparent. A short time after getting her first job, she took driver's education. Much earlier in their lives together, my dad had tried to teach her to drive. It hadn't been successful. Patience wasn't one of his strengths.

One evening at dinner, she laid her new driver's license in the center of the table so we could all see it. My dad was stunned. He had never imagined her driving. But the very next day, he bought her her first car, a yellow Pinto. At age fifty-two she became the woman she had longed to be. What a great example to us, her children. It told me one is never too old. When I turned fifty-two, my life paralleled hers. I took a class to learn how to drive a motorcycle.

It's certain that my generation, our generation, had great role models. It's probable that everyone reading this essay had parents like mine, in some respects, parents who worked hard and expected their children to do likewise. And it's just as probable that your offspring have looked at you like you looked at your parents. Whatever your example was, you have seen it repeated. That's both the good and the bad of our lives as we reflect on them.

Reflection now is serving us in a different way. We have time to explore new beginnings, or pursue, once again, former interests. Some of our dreams have been fulfilled, many of them were deferred, and some may seem farfetched. Dreams are often farfetched, and yet there are philosophers and other lofty-minded people who think that anything we dream has presented itself solely *because it is attainable*. It is *our next goal*, if we dare to grab hold of it. I'm thrilled by this idea, actually. And I hope you are thrilled too. We are simply growing older, we aren't growing dumber. Our personality is still evident in our relationships with others, and our creativity and sensitivity, if anything, are heightened. As we look to our future, we can be confident that whatever our desire may be, our skills for attainment are already honed. Nothing stands in our way but our fear.

As this book's title suggests, to live long and with passion is the gift that's been promised to us if we decide to unwrap it. I have made that choice. I am here, in your life, to help you make that choice too. Are you ready?

Be quiet for a moment. Put this book aside. Empty your mind. As thoughts flutter through your mind (and they will, I assure you), let them escape. Give them their freedom. Breathe, pause, breathe. Now close your eyes. Hear the stillness. Simply sit.

When you feel ready, and only then, write down all the things you have even an inkling to do someday. Every one of them. There are no wrong choices. None at all!

My own list includes the desire to write a novel. It also includes a decision to take a class on writing fiction. I'm excited. I know it's time to take this plunge. And I've invited a friend to take a class too. Having a partner to write with will be my inspiration.

What I suggest you do next is choose two or three dreams and make a plan. Write the steps you think might be necessary to fulfill your dreams. Remember, no idea surfaces that is truly beyond you.

Dream #1:

Dream #2:

Create an affirmation that will help you get started. Write it in your journal.

Tomorrow is the first day of the rest of your life. Your dream is headed your way. Right now. If you doubt this, ask a friend to "hold" the dream for you. Email me and I will hold it too. Send it to karencasey@me.com.

44

Letting Go of the Past

Memories that haunt us into old age are asking to be looked at with fresh eyes. Maybe the time is now.

Digging up the past can be an arduous undertaking. I'm not suggesting that anyone needs to do it. In fact, unless something is bothering you pretty consistently, I'd say leave well enough alone. But if some long-past experience is causing you repeated unease, particularly if it is interfering with your current primary relationships, revisiting the memory is worth considering. Asking someone to revisit it with you might be helpful too. Going into a dark neighborhood alone isn't good at any time. Perhaps your past is far different from mine, but some of my memories were very dark.

Appreciating all that we have learned throughout our life serves us well. It's a spiritually productive awareness, in fact. And I believe that every experience, even those experiences that were particularly unpleasant, those experiences that we strongly resisted, were all part of our necessary learning curve. However, just because they were educational, just because they served our specific development, doesn't mean they didn't occasionally hurt us, at times hurt us deeply. And even though we have learned to celebrate the education we received, old hurts can still gnaw at us. It's time to release them. It's time to be free.

Perhaps it's not clear why I have chosen this topic to explore in a book about passionate living. I might be making an assumption about you, the reader, that's inaccurate. But I can't grab all there is to grab from each moment if something from the past is still wandering around in my mind.

A few years ago that's exactly what was happening to me. The childhood sexual abuse I was forced to experience lived in the shadows of my mind. It had been there for decades. The first few years after it had happened, the memory simply made me sick, and even scared.

As I got older, it made me mad. The anger about it escalated and it impacted all my relationships, particularly those with men. At that time in my life, I wanted to savor the anger. I felt sure I deserved to be angry. And then I knew I had to be done with it. Done with it for good. But how? My process was to write about it. First from my perspective, and then, much to my amazement, from his. I didn't realize when this "inner voice" began to speak that he was calling to me, but indeed, he was. I listened and poured out the words I heard at the computer. Each and every painful utterance. And then it was done. He was done. And I was too. The anger was finished. Forgiveness began to fill the space it left. In time, it filled the entire space.

And then I was free. The experiences in my life felt lighter, more joyful, less serious. It seemed easier to love people, myself included, to accept their shortcomings, and to overlook their errors. I know that had I not given up the anger, I could not have experienced forgiveness in such a complete way. And it was that that changed me. Changed me profoundly.

I began to realize at a much deeper level that my journey, every tiny detail of it, was purposeful. My experience with forgiveness allowed me to share with other women the freedom I felt. I knew, without question, that my childhood experience, though disturbing, was serving other women in a fruitful way. If I could forgive, so could they.

I think the time may be right for you to acknowledge those past experiences which still cling to you. Getting free is mandatory, I think, if you want to fully embrace this next stage of life, a stage of life that I think could be the best stage of all. How it will benefit you and others is directly tied to how free you feel to enjoy whatever activity falls into your lap.

The best way to begin is simply to begin. Here. And now. By collecting and then listing those memories, one by one, that come to mind. Not just any memory, for this assignment, but those memories you don't really want to be troubled by. They can't quit troubling you until you release them. Completely. And then forgive the incidents as well as the perpetrators.

Looking at my past now, this memory rushes toward me . . .

My willingness to let it go is . . .

Is the freedom you feel palpable? Write about it.

Sharing this experience with a trusted friend, or perhaps a counselor, might serve you. Or not. Your wellbeing is what matters. Nothing more. Final thoughts on this newfound freedom.

45

Feeling the Wow

Remembering you are going to die is the best way I know to avoid the trap of thinking you have something to lose. There is no reason not to follow your heart.

—Steve Jobs

I love this quote by Steve Jobs. He surely was a great example for following one's bliss, letting one's heart dictate the journey. Apparently nothing got in his way. Except cancer and then death. Before they interrupted his journey, however, he was driven. He was exceptional, creatively speaking. He pushed others to be exceptional too. It's been reported that his final word, as heard by his wife, as he lay dying, was "wow." Whether or not that's actually true, I don't know. But I want to think it is. I want to believe that passing on to our final home is an experience worthy of the expression "wow." I want to feel the *wowness* of the last stage.

I read a book many years ago on fulfilling your heart's desire while taking a course on spiritual development at a Unity church. It was an amazingly inspirational, hopeful book. I can still remember how motivated I felt about the unfolding of the rest of my life. While it's true I have been faced with a lot of uphill challenges over the years, alcoholism being just one of them, I remained convinced that I was capable of getting through them all.

I was also convinced that my life had purpose, a divine purpose that was specific to me. As a matter of fact, the back cover copy of the book *Illusions* by Richard Bach promised me that in 1977. His words got me over a hump. They stuck with me. They still resonate with me.

I know that writing the many personal growth books that have kept me engaged since the publication of the first one, *Each Day a New Beginning* in 1982, is my way of following my heart, of fulfilling my purpose in the same way as Jobs's creation of Apple was his. Hopefully, you have been following your heart too. It's not too late to begin, however, if you feel that hasn't been your path. Let me guide you in the effort if this challenge is one you want to pursue at long last. This final stage of life is a great time to begin if your calling hasn't yet been fulfilled.

How does one determine their "calling"? How is it recognized? I think you know what it is. I think we always know what's in our hearts. Too often we shy away from it, assuming, perhaps, that it's beyond our reach, that it's arrogant of us to think we can accomplish it. It's here that I want to say, "Stop it!" Whatever is in your mind, no matter how grand it seems to be, is attempting to engage your interest. That it's presenting itself to you can't be denied. What comes to us as a dream is the invitation to tackle it, in fact. All that's left for us to do is make the plan, the step-by-step method of getting there. And even that process will come to us when we seek help from the inner guide who has helped us in other ways our whole life.

There is nothing very mysterious here. It may sound mysterious, but that's only because we haven't acknowledged that's how life has been working all along. Doesn't it give you a sense of wellbeing knowing your course has been charted? That you are fulfilling a specific plan with your name written all over it? If you doubt the truth of this, cast the doubt aside for now. Simply go with the inner inclination and see how it feels to move into the activity that is calling to you. The journey, in due time, will comfort you. Trust me. Please.

Now let's get into the bliss of our lives. Let's take Steve Jobs at his word. Let's feel the "wow" of this life before we even get to the next one. You may not know what to do first. Let me suggest you get quiet. Really quiet. As I suggested early on in this book, breathe, pause, breathe. Close your eyes if that's comfortable. It might be helpful to count backward from one hundred. And then simply sit quietly. After a spell of silence, imagine your spiritual guide coming to meet you. You both sit quietly and then the guide says, "Here's what I think . . . Here's what I can see as your next calling."

Let your heart speak now. Just your heart. Trust what you hear. No matter what you hear. Share it in your journal.

The only thing left to do is make the plan to fulfill the message you received. Why not write it down?

And finally, how does it feel to know where you are going first in this next phase of your life?

Who are you going to tell? Share the plan to make it real. Now.

46

Your Mission Statement

Do you have a mission statement for this stage of life? The idea of having a mission statement for the direction of your life in this latter stage may seem pretty unusual and unnecessary. When the thought first came to me, I chuckled and discarded it. A mission statement? Why? We are more or less retired, aren't we? And then it tugged at me again. Why not create a mission statement? Why not have a specific idea of how to spend all these newly found precious hours, and days, and maybe even years? It is the perfect way to focus our energy, our attention, our resources. Floundering is debilitating. I know. I have done a bit of that of late and I have a major focus: *this book.*

How does one determine a mission statement for retirement, or at least the slowed-down life we deserve to enjoy? Many of us aren't going to fully retire. Ever. I fall into this category, at least for now. I want to work less, however. I have determined that. But I am not interested in withdrawing from the world of ideas and words, or the community of people I spend many weekends with facilitating workshops. I can never walk completely away. Never. But I can regroup and define my life in a way more fitting for me as a seventy-five-year-old woman.

I would love for us to talk over this idea together. But in lieu of that, I want to think out loud about my mission statement and share it with you here. It's my hope that you will be inspired too. Having a direction and a plan ensures that we will find contentment, I believe. At least that's how my past has felt. From the time that I published my first book in 1982, I have had an inkling that grew into a full-blown concept about the second one, the third one, and for every other one too. The one you are holding now is number thirty. I didn't get here with a finely detailed plan. For the most part, it was just a direction. But none of us will go far, ever, without a plan. Even only a sketchy plan is okay. For the purpose of simplicity and familiarity, I'm calling our plan a mission statement.

Mission statement #1: I will continue doing what I have always done since launching my writing and speaking profession. I will simply work far less, and breathe more.

It's my mission to continue reaching out to others, and the most comfortable way for me to do that is to show up at lots of meetings, both AA and Al-Anon, and do a smattering of seminars on the topics that continue to interest me the most: cultivating peaceful relationships and nurturing productive, fulfilling recoveries.

Mission statement #2: I will take a fiction writing class and begin my first novel. For fun. Strictly for fun.

The main difference in what I will be doing is the number of hours I'll commit, daily, to the pursuit. I'm accustomed to spending more than six hours at the computer daily. Some days much longer. And while I have made it clear in other essays that I love what I do and feel called to do it, a slower pace is also calling to me.

———

Now I turn this over to you. Give yourself some breathing room here, meditate for a few minutes if that will help, and then write down, as quickly as possible, that thing you most want to do now that time permits.

Now that you have done that, create an affirmation that states your plan. It will serve as your mission statement, which in turn will pinpoint your direction.

My first mission statement is . . .

Perhaps you are like me and feel drawn to a second mission for this stage of your life. I love reading good fiction and used to be in a short story writing group. I loved it. In fact, I thought my stories were pretty good. However, the *New Yorker* wasn't so impressed. I figured, why not start at the top when trying to get one of them published? I imagine you are chuckling at my naïve arrogance. I am. But it was good practice. Trying fiction again excites me, and that's what any mission for our lives, our spare time, needs to do.

If you have a second goal, bravo! Please describe it in detail. Then tell a friend. That, in itself, will become the first two steps toward the goal's completion.

My second mission statement is . . .

At the end of the day, how does it feel to be moving forward with clear and specific direction? It brings me a sense of relief. It comforts me to know my life remains purposeful.

47

Shape Your Mind

Our life is shaped by our mind. We become what we think.

—Buddha

This isn't a new idea to any of us, I'm sure. But laziness prevents us from keeping our minds under our control, thus on a path that is beneficial to others, as well as ourselves. Instead, we wander into neighborhoods that may be dark, certainly unproductive, and peopled with naysayers to whom we give control over our thoughts. Before we know it, our thoughts begin to mimic their thoughts, and we become strangers to who we really want to be.

This describes my earlier experiences to a T. Until 1971, when I read a significant passage in a book by John Powell, a passage that asked, "Why should I let him decide what kind of day I'm going to have?" my life had always been a reflection of what *your thoughts were*, at times a reaction to them; at other times their mirror image. What was always the case: my thoughts were never my very own. Never.

If this dilemma has tripped you up in the past, it really doesn't have to hold sway over you now, or ever again. Hallelujah! In our youth, I think we were far more susceptible to influences that were not beneficial. We wanted to be liked, to fit in, to be on the list of the chosen few. Chosen for what didn't much matter. Just chosen!

When I was young, the group I especially wanted to want me was "the superlatives." And I made it in. What a boost to my ego it was when I put the chain around my neck, a chain with a silver scroll hanging from it. The scroll was inscribed with an Old English S. My ego began to lead me astray almost immediately, and continued to pull me in a direction that ran counter to who I now prefer being. I was hostage to my ego. But what I can say now, with confidence, is that my journey, every step of it, was necessary for the honing my persona needed. I wouldn't be *here,* with all of you, without having been *there. Every single there!* This I know for sure.

Perhaps others held you hostage in the past too. Other people or other circumstances often have that power over us. Of course, we have relinquished our own power, and quite willingly too. Being fully responsible for every circumstance of one's life is a bitter pill to swallow. Alas. But I don't mean for this essay to be a downer. On the contrary. Discovering that we were and are the sole deciders about our life is quite empowering.

It's also a heavy burden initially. At least emotionally. The good news is this: just as quickly as we learned we were accountable, in fact, had to be accountable, we also learned we could change every idea we held, every action we were contemplating, every dream we were nurturing about the future we had yet to claim.

Everything, absolutely everything, all experiences, every person, each and every dream, is moving us toward better tomorrows. If that's what we have our sights on. *If . . .* What's especially wonderful about this idea is that aging, which is where we so comfortably rest currently (if that's our mindset), can be faced with healthy anticipation. Excitement even. Or a soft, secure quietness. One thing we need never feel is dread. Never dread.

Because I want to be honest with all of you, and as authentic as I've always tried to be in the past in all my books and workshops, I have to say my own reach into the future, my own thoughts about how the next few years might look, have created in me a feeling of uneasiness that I don't want to admit to. If I didn't consider all of you as friends, perhaps friends I have yet to meet, but friends anyway, I wouldn't be able to admit this. After all, I am the author of the book you are now reading. Shouldn't I have mastered my suggestions to you in my own life first?

Perhaps I should have. You may well think so too. But it's really not unusual, I think, to live a principle well one day and completely forget it the following day. The ego works overtime in its effort to trip us up. And yet I have come to see this circumstance in a positive light. Whenever the ego throws me off course, I become even more determined to cling to the spiritual voice that wants so very much to be heard.

To reiterate one of my fondest beliefs, a belief that right-sizes me in a nanosecond: we have two voices in our minds. One is always peaceful, loving, and directing us to act in ways consistent with love. The other voice is directly opposite to that. Never a peaceful moment will be experienced if the ego is in charge. You can easily determine which voice I have listened to of late. But I am now right-sized again. Just talking about it, not keeping it a secret, has released me from its hold.

Let's get down to the business at hand. Here we are, you and I, on a journey that promises fulfillment into our advanced years, and my conversations with folks from all walks of life are resoundingly similar on one thing: being fulfilled is what we are looking for. The only thing required of us is to decide what will create our fulfillment. Is it by doing something specific? Maybe volunteering at a shelter, an elementary school, a nursing home, or a senior center, perhaps? Or is it by simply offering a loving response every moment we have with another human being?

Our choices are many. The only thing that feels necessary is to make one. Eventually. Some of us will want to continue working, at least part-time. That's where I'll find my fulfillment. In fact, this book is serving as my fulfillment at the present time. Although I'm seventy-five and counting, I am not counting on ever quitting, on sitting down and saying, "That's all folks, I'm done." In fact, over lunch today I told a friend I already had an idea for my next book. And it felt so good to own that.

Enough from me. It's time for you to search out your mind. I'm hopeful that my meanderings will give you the latitude you need for your search. And perhaps these questions will draw you in to discovering your heart's pure desire. That's where your next activity resides.

Questions:

1. What was your favorite activity while in grade school? High school? College?

2. Is there any interest in pursuing that activity again? Or a related activity?

3. How might it look?

4. If you are beginning this phase of your life from scratch, make a list of the activities outside work that have interested you since your profession got off the ground. Some of you maybe joined a bridge group, a tennis club, a writing group, or took on volunteer activities because you were expected to by your employer. List all of them and recreate how doing them now might look. Any interest building?

This is not about making busywork for yourselves. This is about finding yourselves all over again, seeing who you could be now that you have the time to recreate yourself. Dare to be brave. The sky is the limit. I have a friend who decided at age sixty and after recovering from lung cancer to run a 5K race in every state in the union. She accomplished that. Her next goal is to break a racing record at the Bonneville Salt Flats running a '49 Ford pickup with an original flat-head engine. It's my guess that she will succeed.

It's not about choosing a grand goal. Just one that will captivate you.

One of my goals for you is that you enjoy the search. This can best be assured if you refuse to be limited by your thinking. Simply assume you can do or accomplish anything that comes to mind. Why? You can! Trust me. Now close your eyes and imagine yourself engaged. How does it feel? What is engaging you?

In closing this essay, I'd like to encourage you to share what you are undertaking with a friend who is treading water. He or she needs some direction. Your experience, coupled with your success and commitment, paints for her the picture she needs to put one foot in front of the other. Share in your journal what you will share with her.

The universe changes when we change how we interact with the universe. It begins in the family. It moves to the community and the workplace, the library, or the movie theater next. The grocery store, the lanes of traffic, the total strangers we pass on the streets are not to be discounted. It's called the butterfly effect when we name that which modifies the other side of the world with each action you or I take. *Wow!* It's for real. Let's celebrate it. Let's double up on our efforts now that we have time to recreate ourselves. What's the first change you will make today? Envision how it might impact others.

Are you happy now that life is changing? Describe who you see in the mirror when you get up.

What's on your gratitude list on a regular basis now?

What can you imagine will be on your gratitude list now that you are heading in a new, exciting direction?

———————————

48

Overcoming Fear

A man's true delight is to do the things he was made for.
—Marcus Aurelius

I will admit to an occasional slip of the mind. I'm not perfect, after all. I had one slip recently, in fact. My husband and I were discussing some of our plans for the next phase of our lives: where we might live when we can no longer drive, how to continue managing two homes, quite likely making the decision to give up one, but which one? And then live where? Surprisingly, we were not on the same page, which isn't a common occurrence. Realizing that resulted in my becoming fearful. A space I hadn't lived in for some time. Nothing he said helped.

Of course we got it sorted out. Neither of us likes to be discomforted, but it surprised me just how quickly I forgot everything I know to be true—every tool, every principle, every cherished idea I so commonly "preach" in my books and workshops. I was even more surprised by the fear that overwhelmed me. I had not felt that degree of fear for years. Was there an additional underlying reason for my reaction? Perhaps. Turning seventy-five is a big deal. Putting the wheels in motion for a less busy life created my need for an adjustment. I felt uneasy in an interesting way. I'm not used to feeling uneasy.

In addition to our discussion about our future, each year our return to Minnesota from Naples, Florida, puts my psyche in a tizzy until I get everything nailed down in my study. I have to sink my feet into who I am, no matter where I am. When I am on the road, I think I lose sight of that. The road trip has a sense of homelessness about it. And I'm a homebody.

What my unexpected experience with fear also showed me, and the reason I am sharing it with you, is that any transition in our lives can be unsettling. And having a big birthday, coupled with the move back to Minnesota, plus the discussion about the future, a future I'm not ready to look at, flipped me into a space where I felt untethered. Being untethered, even for a few hours, reminded me of the abyss I stared into after a year of recovery. It was a scary place, and then, as now, I couldn't grab on to anything for security. This circumstance was short-lived, but profoundly powerful. Our minds, when ruled by the ego, can scare the heck out of us. I know. I've just been there.

But the good news about getting through a fearful situation like this is that we know we can get through it again, and again, if need be. The circumstances of life are ever-changing. Always. And many of the changes throw us off guard. Fear may be the first response then. Fortunately it's not the only response, or the final response. Mostly we flow with the changes. But when we don't, remembering that this too will pass is a place to begin. All we need is a thread of an idea to hang on to, and it will weave us back into the tapestry that had previously comforted us.

Like I said way back in the introduction, breathe, pause, and breathe again. Even if you are not in a place of gripping fear (and it's not likely that many of you are there), but are simply experiencing a modicum of uncertainty, pause for a moment to remember what we have been promised: that everything that's happening, that will ever happen, or did happen was *never* unorchestrated. God was always the conductor. However, you were the first chair. Co-creation was in the symphony being played. And that's a big deal. Just like turning seventy-five is a big deal.

Reflecting on who we really are, in the midst of change, opens the door to being willing to comfort ourselves if that's what's needed. You are facing a changing future, one that will never be stationary, in fact. Aging requires us to recognize that. Quite possibly that's what drew you to this book. Like my life, yours no longer requires a forty- or fifty-hour workweek. And fear might befriend you now. That's okay. She needs to know you will not abandon her, but will walk her through every moment of change that comes. The idea of befriending our fear is designed to comfort us. And while it comforts, it also helps us release the fear. It doesn't need us for a home. We are too busy creating a space for our next chapter.

Fear may be a visitor at your door. But you don't have to embrace it. Simple acknowledgment is quite enough. It's not looking for a celebration. It's just looking for comfort too. Keep your sights on what your dream is now. What lights the fire within you? Something heretofore untried? Or a refinement of an already well-practiced skill? It matters not. What counts is that it will bring joy to you because that's what will spread joy to others too.

Life before the afterlife is the stage we are experiencing now. Making it rich and rewarding is what I'm hoping for. My guess is that's what you are hoping for too. But we need a plan. We need a destination, and by that I don't mean a new location. We simply need to know when we get up every morning the direction we are heading that day. Are we volunteering or are we working part-time? Are we at a painting class or teaching a writer's group? There is no right plan, no one destination. Just the plan and the destination that calls excitedly to you.

If you were to get your fondest dream fulfilled about your future, what would it look like? Tell me yours and then tell someone else about it. I will share mine too.

What I expect for my life has been stated earlier, but it's already become more focused since I first mentioned it. After taking a class in fiction writing from The Loft, I will publish a book of fiction. Either a novel or a book of short stories. I will continue to write recovery and spiritual growth books too. In fact, my next one in that genre will stress the principles I have gleaned from studying *A Course in Miracles* for thirty years. My time will be far freer, since I will be doing far fewer programs for the public. Travel is going to be curtailed. And it feels good having come to that conclusion.

Full-blown retirement does not call to me. I recognize that I have a need to be needed. Writing will more than adequately fulfill that need.

What is calling to you? How will you answer the call? Share the picture of your life in detail in your journal.

What's been the best part of looking into the future?

What has unsettled you or made you feel fearful?

What do you know you must do before it's too late?

49

A Vital Person

We're not on our journey to save the world but to save ourselves. But in doing that you save the world. The influence of a vital person vitalizes.

—Joseph Campbell

The journey of every person reading this is uniquely vital to the world we share. That statement may seem a bit farfetched and a gross exaggeration. But according to the dictionary, vital means valuable and essential. Can every person really be defined this way? For instance, how could Adolf Hitler's journey, the philosophy that led to his actions, his very being, have been considered valuable except to his mother? He certainly wasn't valuable to seven million Jews.

And what about Joseph Stalin, who massacred more than twice the number killed by Hitler? Valuable? Essential? And then there are our own soldiers who have gone a bit crazy in combat, in every war. Hundreds, maybe thousands of innocent civilians have been killed by them. What's so vital, so essential, about those journeys? Perhaps we fail to understand just what Campbell means by "vital." Or maybe we do, and feel so numb by the "vital" actions of some that we can't put our thoughts into words.

But all that aside, I have grown to agree that every heart that beats is beating in a body that is essential. Every mind that thinks, or not, is in a body that counts. My own spiritual journey has convinced me of that. No one is unessential. *Everyone is necessary to the whole of humankind.* Everyone. We simply can't know all the necessary connections being made between any two or more journeying bodies that helped to knit together the tapestry comprising the universe. We simply know it has been woven together. In a perfect way, as a matter of fact.

We are certain our part in this process is a small part. And that may be true. Size is irrelevant, however. Crucial parts of an airplane engine might be almost too small for the naked eye to see, but if one of them is missing, the plane goes down. We can't measure vitality by size. Nor can we measure it by any specific action.

The quote of Campbell's reminds me of one of Margaret Mead's that I have always loved: "Never doubt that a small group of thoughtful, committed citizens can change the world. Indeed, it is the only thing that ever has." Individuals, or collectives who are like-minded, can wield a powerful influence. Each one of us has influence too. Each one of us is undeniably vital. Each activity any one of us engages in is influencing all other activities in that very same moment of time. No action is sacrosanct. We each are particles in the universe of particles, and we are influencing one another constantly; it's referred to as the butterfly effect.

What a profound life we live. Our every moment is impacting every single moment in every other person's life. It's truly mind-boggling. And some think that the life we have yet to live is the most awesome part of all. How enticing this idea is. Wouldn't you say?

I suggest we all step back for a moment and absorb the truth of our existence and the vital, specific ways we affect one another constantly, even though we are oblivious to most of it.

How do you feel, now, after a few moments of contemplation?

We are never not in communication with other souls, even though words aren't always exchanged. There is no separation between us. Ever. We are One. We are One with the universe. We are One with the Creator. We are One with each other, the plants, the trees, the fish in the oceans. It's impossible that we are not in constant communication with all life. We are part of the proverbial all. Now and always. Who are you currently unknowingly influencing, do you suppose?

What a wild thought. Yet what a powerful truth. Just resonating on the oneness that we are, that we share, that we have shared and will always share takes my breath away. Does it take yours away too?

Let's take a moment to reflect.

Who influenced you this morning?

Who was your major influence throughout your career, if you worked outside the home?

And who looked to you as a role model?

Were you a proud, compassionate one?

Did you guide him or her lovingly? In what specific ways?

As we move into this next stage of life, perhaps nurturing this idea of being vital for others can be cultivated as the primary activity we'll engage in. Or through exploring specific activities like playing bridge, gardening, helping an even older elder, singing in a choir, or tutoring young people who have fallen behind. One activity might gain your full attention, deciding for you what comes next now that you have more time. Some know, without a doubt, what the latter stage of life will look like. I do, more or less.

It's not mandatory to know, however. Many will know only that they are ready to slow down and live quietly. Living more lovingly is a good bet too. We will speak more slowly and quietly to our loved ones. We will spend more time just listening. We will ask folks to share their memories and dreams, rather than being the one who always talks.

On the one hand, this may not seem like a big change. On the other hand, it seems huge. I heard a wonderful acronym a few years ago. And it's a great one to practice at any age: WAIT, Why Am I Talking? Silence is a great target to shoot for. At any age, but at this age in particular. Let others tell you about themselves. You have time to listen. Don't you?

Let's not only not talk for now, but let's also not even think for the present time. Instead, let's withdraw and meditate. Simply breathe, pause, and breathe again. Shhhhh . . . Who do you imagine yourself becoming now that you have the time, the inclination, and the sacred willingness to just be?

What a joy to watch me now. My face and eyes tell the world about my happiness, my peace of mind, and my under-standing of the way life works. When we surrender our plan to our Creator, we see with new eyes. We see a new world. We aren't who we used to be. We are transformed. Our perspectives are transformed. Who we show up as in this world has been transformed. What an unexpected gift to carry into this latter stage of life.

Questions to reflect on in our transformed state:

Who will I affect the most?

What will our exchanges look like?

What's the primary addition to my daily gratitude list?

What do I most want others to know about me now?

What do I most want others to know about how I see myself now?

If I'm not content, what do I imagine will content me?

_____

50

Cultivating Warm Relations

The best of conversations occur when there is no competition, no vanity, but a calm quiet interchange of sentiments.

—Samuel Johnson

I love this quote by Johnson. It echoes the kind of conversations I'm accustomed to having now that I'm in the latter, and for many reasons better, stage of life. We do finally reach a place where we don't have to "win" a discussion. In my youth, and perhaps in yours too, discussions were always about making someone else see that my understanding of an idea was the correct interpretation. Hours were wasted in making points that no one cared about, points that didn't matter. Points that were exaggerated most of the time beyond recognition.

It's fortuitous, I think, that as we age, most of us are far more interested in cultivating warm relations with one another. Being constantly agitated loses its luster in time. I speak of what I know. I was the proverbial agitator in my family of origin. I continued carrying that tradition for a number of years, even after I no longer wanted to be angry. I actually didn't know how to change such a well-honed habit. It wasn't until I learned that agitation was equated with fear that I was able to see how to let it go. I had learned this trait at the feet of the master. My dad. He was riddled with fear. Since childhood. He passed it on to me and I glorified it. Until I no longer saw the glory in it.

Since seeing truth, since living in a more peaceful body, I am inclined to share with others what I've come to cherish. Perhaps I'm still trying to influence others to see with my eyes, but the view is pleasant, at least.

I think all of us reach maturity with a set of core beliefs that guide our choices and define our actions. Because of my addiction to alcohol and other drugs, coupled with my extreme codependency, I delayed my maturity. I'd have to say, in fact, that even though I have had no alcohol or taken any drugs for nearly forty years, I wasn't free of the ramifications of codependency until well into my recovery. And being completely honest with you, I still have an occasional codependency relapse. My meltdown, while my husband and I were trying to sort out the next few years of our lives, testifies to that.

The difference is that a meltdown doesn't define the relationship for all time. It's acknowledged, discussed, resolved, amends are made, and the parties move on. Generally. It took a long time to get to this stage of trust, but that's the stuff of relationships. I think. When they are meaningful (and I personally think that each relationship is meaningful to one degree or another, or it wouldn't have developed at all), the teaching and learning that's exchanged is crucial to both parties, if they are to be who they were born to be.

I have said in many places, other essays, and certainly in other books too, that we seek out our learning partners here on planet Earth. We knew before we were born who we'd find. And we knew what the lesson would be. However, we forget both of these facts, so that when someone rattles our cage, we react with fear. That describes to a T how I was the day of my meltdown. My husband and I were not on the same page regarding our future plans. I had not realized our scripts were different. And I got scared. Everything I knew to be true, including the fact that God was part of the solution, was pitched out the window. I wallowed in fear. Until I was done. Until I remembered the ego had run away with me.

We have all been privy to those discussions others are having that seem not to be leading to any solution. And maybe they will peter out with no solution in sight. But one of the tools we can put to use when we are sitting on the sidelines at these times (and we are there by design, remember), is to *hold the parties up to the light.* Say a quiet prayer for them to be open to the ideas of others. And then say the same prayer for ourselves that we may be able to do the same thing the next time we are on opposing sides of an issue.

Our "work" is never done as long as we are alive. We are always needed for one task or another. We are needed wherever we are every minute of the day, in fact. Isn't that a glorious realization?

51

What Are You Grateful for Today?

As a change of pace, I decided that asking a question might stir up some soul searching that would or could move you in a new direction for this last quarter of purposeful living. Don't misunderstand, however. I'm not assuming that you need to switch directions. But we sometimes get into a rut without even realizing it. Until a question like the one I posed here is asked, we blithely trudge along, seldom veering off course, sticking with the choices we have been making for years, not daring to try anything really new for fear of failure. When we are caught in that frame of mind, gratitude is seldom on the radar screen. Having a list of things we are grateful for is certainly not on our screen.

But I'm pushing you to put it on your radar screen for the purpose of this exercise. And you may be surprised. Your list may surprise you. It may go on for pages if you are painstaking about it, or you may discover there is not a lot that comes to mind. Perhaps everything on the list falls into the same category. Some gratitude lists consist only of names of people, rather than activities or achievements. A gratitude list with only names might suggest that other people are more central to your life than you are. There is no right way or wrong way to compile a gratitude list. However, what pleases you about your life should be there. Period.

My own gratitude list includes both people and experiences. I have met some extremely interesting people. One person I am thrilled to call a friend is Bill Moyers. He has given so much to so many through his work in public television, and in the field of addictions too. He paid me a great compliment in a very public forum about my work as a recovery writer, and I've been forever grateful. I'm grateful to have friends who love movies and discussing them, who love playing bridge and golf too. I'm grateful for my husband, Joe. He is fun, creative, supportive, and my best friend.

I'm grateful for my first husband too. Our marriage didn't work, but its failure pushed me into graduate school and my PhD, a degree I had never considered getting, never even imagined I could get, in fact. I'm also grateful that I have become willing to make amends in my life. That has brought me closer to other people, and it has taught me about humility.

Whatever makes its way to our gratitude list is the direct result of a choice we have made. Many of our choices were convenient ones because they accommodated others too. In my age group, and I'm assuming many of you reading this are in my age group too, it was quite common to put the needs of others before our own. There is nothing inherently wrong with that. In many instances it was the obvious choice anyway, and certainly the kindest. However, making choices that benefit others more than ourselves can lead to resentments. And resentments clutter up a potentially peaceful mind. Has this happened to you?

It's been my experience with resentments that they eat away the joy that my life deserves. They can also interfere with something or some person that might have been so lucky as to end up on a gratitude list too. The best way to address resentments is to own them, and as quickly as possible seek through prayer and meditation to let them go so they don't infect any other experiences. When we measure them against our myriad reasons for gratitude, they lose their hold on us pretty quickly.

At the top of my gratitude list is my love of writing. I love it because I sense that someone else is sharing the stage with me, and that comforts me. I feel like I am doing the work that's been chosen for me. I do it with ease, which further suggests that I'm doing the right work. There are so many writing avenues open to me, and that pleases me. I will incorporate a new one for this last stage of life. I'm thinking it will be fiction. I dipped my toes into fiction a few years ago and loved it. Returning to it for pleasure, and only pleasure, will be fun. However, my interest in being published is such that I may not be able to keep it just for fun. Choose something on your gratitude list for exploration now.

If you don't actually pursue the list item you choose in a serious way, just making the choice here is perfectly okay. What you are doing is practicing for the final stage, the final exam, so to speak. I think it's fair to say that we all want to go out with a sense of wellbeing, the sense that we did what was expected of us, that we didn't disappoint the God of our understanding. I'm certain that no matter how we performed, we didn't disappoint.

Let's begin that gratitude list now. Before we forget about it. Begin with people. Who are those people who have meant so much to you over your life? Who helped to guide you when you were young? How about your teen years? During and after college? Your first real job? The career you settled on, or at least the one you went for initially?

When it comes to family life, was there someone who helped you figure out the kind of spouse you were seeking? How about the direction you wanted to go in when it came time to raise a family? So many individuals pass through our lives. Many of them leave a deeply indelible mark, even though they are only present for a short time. Do you have any people like this you want to put on the list?

Significant decisions need to be remembered, as well as the people who helped you make them. Putting them down on paper is a way of reminding yourself that you may want to drop them a note of thanks, even if their help was offered a number of years ago. It's never too late to remember a good deed. No one is ever offended by a thank-you note.

Let's go next to the experiences that impacted you. Those that still hold sway over your mind and your current decision-making. You may find, like I have found, that patterns of behavior were developed years ago as the result of a particular experience. Being grateful for the experience is good for one's soul. It's also a way of acknowledging our Higher Power, who I believe was always in on the experience. Life is intentional. Always. Every experience was on the chart. Always. The people we have met were selected by us. Always. Putting the names and experiences down on paper where we can visualize them once again is a lovely way to say thank you before we move on to stage four.

And now let's explore the past.

The people . . .

The experiences . . .

The impact . . .

What goes forth with me now?

I know my life has been well lived because . . .

Do You Like Yourself Enough?

Perhaps this strikes you as an odd question in a book like this; however, time is running out. I write this assuming you are over sixty years old (perhaps not seventy-five like yours truly). Liking ourselves at any age is crucially important, in my opinion. Falling into the state of dislike is so common when we are youngsters (a pandemic, currently, one might say), and unfortunately, many of us grew up in families that were riddled with dysfunction, making our low self-esteem a common theme, one that has led to suicide by youngsters far too often.

The good news is that it's never too late to recast who we are and how we feel about ourselves, and others too. In my case, it took recovery from alcoholism to clarify where my demons were and how to transform them into allies. Having a dad who was so riddled with fear that he'd make a mistake, made living up to his expectations nearly impossible. None in our family were unscathed, feeding his failure even more.

Our family of origin left a deep and indelible mark on who we were, how we perceived the world we lived in, and, quite unfortunately, defined the footprint we were going to leave as we wandered, sometimes downtrodden, through life. "Wherever we go, there we are," is a cliché with more than just a faint ring of truth to it. And we will, or we did, bring into adulthood that person we were influenced to be as a youngster sitting at the kitchen table. Most of us weren't strong enough to dodge the bullets that were flying, bullets that demeaned us even though they were shot from a gun that actually defined the shooter.

I feel fortunate, very grateful in fact, to have developed alcoholism in my teens. Even though I didn't get into recovery from it until my mid-thirties, I did get the tools there that not only allowed me to gradually become the woman I was meant to be, but also revealed so much about the parents *I had chosen* as mine. The education I got from using those tools also helped me express the love my parents truly deserved. They did the best they could. I came to an appreciation of this, which I'm so grateful for. The tools also informed me about my place in their lives, in the lives of all the people I encountered throughout my lifetime, and they have fully prepared me to be grateful for all the experiences that are yet to come.

I dare to suggest to you that even though alcoholism might not have been part of your journey (probably wasn't, in fact), whatever you did experience, however you did see yourself, the people who showed up on your path were all there *as invited*. Let me emphasize this last statement: *as invited*. And if your self-esteem was hindered by those encounters, as mine was, that too served the purpose of propelling you forward. And here we are, in a late stage of life, having an opportunity to become who we still want to be, to do what we still want to do, and to fulfill any dreams that still continue calling to us. How much better can it get? And yet, to do any of this, it will help if we like ourselves in the way we deserve to like ourselves.

Perhaps it seems too self-serving to you to "work" to like yourself more. And I certainly don't want to presume you don't like yourself right now. But in my seventy-five years, I have yet to meet a man or woman who hasn't expressed a wish that they were happier with their accomplishments, happier with their place in life, better at some activity, or certain that the future held for them a special gift as yet unopened. For some, having a desire to do something quite out of the realm of what they have done in the past might be noodling around in the mind.

I can make a list of many activities I intend to explore after I quit being a road warrior. I have loved my work, still do in fact, but my body doesn't love the travel as much as it used to. Perhaps offering workshops online will be one avenue for me. I can't fathom no longer writing. That certainly won't happen. Writing is in my bones. It's in my DNA. It's my direct line of communication with the spirit world. And I don't say that lightly. I know that when I sit before a screen with my hands poised over the keyboard, that's my invitation to the inner voice to offer the words that want to be heard. I am on call. Always on call.

I also want to explore the genre of fiction more seriously. I mentioned in an earlier essay the short story group I was in a decade ago, and I know I want to revisit that form of writing. It pleased me to be pulled forward by characters that simply appeared in my head. I also have tried watercolors in years past. Acrylics is where I want to go next. Abstracts I think. But most of all, I want to explore silence and the gift of doing nothing. I want to make sure I am not putting plans on my chart titled What to Do Next just so I won't feel my life has lost value. I want to feel my value even when I offer nothing new to the world. I don't think I can get there without some new practices. Prayer and meditation are high on that list. But also on the list is silence. Simply silence. Not even meditating, just the moment-by-moment joy of silence that I think awaits me. I haven't trusted to go there yet, however. It's time is coming.

I think it may be easier for us to move into this need do nothing stage if we celebrate, ever so quietly, all that we have done that has brought us to this new plateau. On my list are: a bachelor's degree from Purdue University; eight years as a successful elementary teacher; being part of an experimental teachers' group in St. Paul, Minnesota that used only positive reinforcement in a summer school program with at-risk kids to test what gets children to desire success; both a master's degree and a PhD in American Studies from the University of Minnesota; my work at Hazelden Foundation; my service on their board for nine years; my thirty books (and counting) published. All of these make me very proud. I assure you, your list is long as well. And although I'm not proud of my alcoholism, I am grateful for it because it led me to many of my successes, not the least of which are the PhD and the publication of thirty books.

Your turn.

Included among my collection of successes are the following (now, don't be afraid to pat yourself on the back!) . . .

The possibilities that call to me right now about how the future might look are many and varied. Those I favor most are . . .

To conclude this essay, I want to say that the choices we have made over the decades we have lived were perfect for us. Each and every one of them needed to be experienced by us. We set up our lives before we were born. I have mentioned this concept in earlier essays, and you may not be entirely on board with it. I wasn't when I was first introduced to it. But it has brought me peace to believe it. A tremendous amount of peace, and at our age, that's what we deserve, after all. It's my guess that you might agree with that too.

53

Your Mind Holds the Power

To love and be loved, one must do good to others. The inevitable condition whereby to become blessed, is to bless others.

—Mary Baker Eddy

Mary Baker Eddy is considered the founder of the Christian Science movement, a movement that asserts that illness is an illusion and healing is fostered through prayer. Her belief and commitment to healing through prayer is an idea that holds sway even today in the lives of thousands. I am not suggesting in this essay that we should necessarily make a commitment to this belief system. On the contrary, I suggest only that the power of the mind, your mind and mine, is beyond our wildest imagination. And that's the good news.

Of course, through the mind I can also create many unwanted problems. It's the latter that is unfortunately the most common for many of us. We live chaotic, painful lives because they directly reflect, project some would say, *what's in our minds.*

We arrived here, however, to this stage of life, and our minds were solely in charge, whether we acknowledged that or not. Because of this we can safely assume, I think, that we can chart where we go next in the very same manner. "As I think, so I am," to paraphrase René Descartes. Running with this idea at any age determines our direction, defines our accomplishments, decides our fate. That's an idea that is to be cherished. At least by this septuagenarian. Wouldn't you agree?

Our minds are in charge. Taking this perspective as our mindset for explaining a past we might have been confused about, the present which is still very much ours to determine, and the persona we will forge to experience the future we can still design, gives us forward momentum. And then to roll this realization into Mary Baker Eddy's quote underscores the importance of giving away to others only that which we'd like to receive in return. We are never too old to consciously paint the life we still want to experience by observing very carefully our actions, our attitudes, and our opinions. Each one of them has sculpted who we were, and is still sculpting who we are, and thus what we will receive in turn from others. What fun, really, to have this much control over how one's life unfolds.

One way to collect all that this has meant in the past is to look carefully at both peak experiences and struggles that are now long over, for the opportunity to see them more objectively, thus more clearly, than ever before. This inventory of those experiences that come most quickly to mind is a great teaching device. I assure you, we do not forget those that did the most to define us in that time and place. As a matter of fact, every previous experience was defining us. Every one of them. The same will hold sway throughout our remaining years on this planet. That's very good news. It assures us that we still have a chance, in fact millions of chances most likely, to forge who we will be within every experience. Every one of them. What has been true before, in this regard, will never change.

My peak experiences that scream out to be remembered are . . .

The struggles that nearly did me in were . . .

The overview of your past, as you have just done, is all the evidence you need, I think, to design how you want your future to look, particularly when it has become your past. Our minds are all powerful. This is true whether we are adherents of the Christian Science belief system or not. We can't change truth. Ever. And what is true now and always will be true is that our perspectives, thus our minds, determine who we see, what we see, thus who we become in the moment, each moment, as we live it.

We too seldom take conscious advantage of that. But there is no time like the present to change how we consciously live.

Beginning right now, who do you want others to see, to experience, when they are with you? Take a few moments to quiet your mind and then "draw" with words who this person is.

How does it feel to know, in a very active way, that you are in charge, solely in charge, of who you introduce to each moment? In order to see this for yourself, create a brief scenario that reflects an encounter between you and a loved one that reveals who you truthfully are.

Now do the same exercise, but it's an encounter with a stranger.

You are the one in charge. You have always been in charge. You will remain in charge for as long as you live. I'd suggest that every one of us should consider giving this last stage of our lives to benefitting the universe in a positive way. It's waiting for us. The tipping point to the attainment of a truly peaceful world is just a moment away. You and I have the power to make anything we want happen. You and I.

_____

54

Random Acts of Fun

Random acts of kindness can make the difference that truly matters. Have you performed one lately? I remember when I read the little book *Random Acts of Kindness* that was published in 2002 by Conari Press. I loved the simplicity of the book. I loved the idea inherent in it. And I loved the accessibility of performing tiny, kind acts on a whim. I continue to think it's the kind of idea that can sweep a community, even shift the universe, if the tipping point is reached.

I also love that Conari has been my publisher for more than a handful of books in the last decade. Being a respected author of recovery, self-help, and spiritual growth books since the publication of *Each Day a New Beginning* in 1982 has given my life steady focus, profound joy, and such an easy way to live my passion. It's definitely my intention to stay on this same path in one genre or another until I can write no more. That pronouncement thrills me. And that day will never come, I imagine.

I remember seeing the movie, *Frida*, produced in 2002, which traced the life of the painter Frida Kahlo. She was a renowned, though somewhat eccentric, Mexican painter who was married to Diego Rivera. Her commitment to her art never wavered, and I admired that. In fact, when she could no longer stand because of the pain of a shattered back, she lay on her side and continued painting, ignoring her circumstances. I marveled at her passion for her work, work she simply had to do. And I feel a kinship to her passion.

It's my conjecture that every one of us felt, in the past (and the lucky ones among us still feel it in the present), an inner passion for work that we did or are still doing, or for some other activity that consumed us in a good way. Maybe we volunteered as a mentor for a young man or woman who was trying to figure out how to network, how to choose a major for college, or how to sort through their life experiences so they could be highlighted in a résumé.

Activities that sparked the inner flame of real joy are to be cherished and perhaps even resurrected for these times of less intense busyness. We won't be the only ones to benefit if we do this. Whatever good works we do for one are actually being done for everyone, everywhere. Remember my earlier references to the butterfly effect?

To have the freedom now, as so many of us have, to make good choices about how to spend our remaining years, even how to spend the hours of any one day, is such a blessing, one we can be grateful for every day that we have left.

It's not my intention to be maudlin here. On the contrary, I consider it a plus to review lives well lived. It's even more of a plus to still be living our lives in the lane marked "fulfilling." We can keep the list of fulfilling experiences going if we listen to our hearts. They always know what's pleasing. They always know when we are spending our hours in worthy ways. There is no more worthy way than to do unannounced random acts of kindness and sit back and watch the world around you respond. No one is unaffected. No one!

Keeping this idea, this potential action, in the ready to implement mode means we always have something fun on the horizon to do. Keeping the passion alive in our lives doesn't take major planning. It doesn't mean we have to do anything in particular. Just be at the ready to offer up a kindness to an unsuspecting person. Lately some person in San Francisco, and another one in St. Louis too, has been leaving clues and hiding money in various locations all over the city. They are not seeking notoriety. They are remaining anonymous, in fact. They are simply sharing their wealth. The joy is experienced by both the givers and the finders. The joy is palpable, and it seems contagious. Contagious in a very good way.

Making a difference in the life of another person is what I'm suggesting here. Perhaps there is no greater way to experience a sense of connection, of wellbeing than making life a tiny bit better for someone else. We have all known people who are stingy. And generally, they had personalities that matched. We didn't seek them out, did we? Their lack of generosity affected every part of their behavior. Joy was in short supply when we were with them.

The main point of this essay is simply to suggest we have more fun before our time on this planet runs out. Make it the primary objective during these remaining years. None of us can guess, with anything like certainty, the moment that will be our last. Perhaps some among us have been diagnosed recently with a terminal condition. The doctor may have even said that it's likely death will come in three to six months. But he or she doesn't really know. All medical predictions are based on guesses, some good guesses, but most not so good. The one thing I know to be correct is that our last breath won't be taken until our myriad assignments on this plane have been completed.

Not knowing when that last breath will be taken is actually a great motivator to live larger. Live fully now. Live as though this very day is your last. How do you really want to spend it? Whom do you want to be with? Your legacy is still being created. Don't squander these moments, these opportunities, these encounters with the remaining individuals who have been charted to meet with you. They deserve their time with you. You deserve every breath you need to take in their presence.

I'm hoping this essay finds a special place in your heart. We discount ourselves so much, I fear. And time is running out for us to acknowledge, with pride coupled with humility, who we have been, how we have shown up on the path bearing our name. Just as was true of our parents, we did our best along the way. We hit the wall a few times. We offered lousy guidance on occasion. We failed to fulfill a number of our very achievable goals, and there is no shame in that. We can fill many pages with the good stuff we did manage to achieve. And that's what I want you to do now. Focus on the good stuff! Write it down. Look at it closely. Thank your God for all the help you received in order to claim each and every item on the list.

Begin now. My good stuff is here for me to celebrate. For me to share with others if I so choose.

And in the time remaining, I hope to add some or all of the following activities to my list of good stuff.

What a life! So much to be grateful for. Praise be to the source of all inspiration.

55

Expressing Thanks

What piece of advice did you receive from a parent or grandparent that still lingers in your memory? Did you ever take the time to tell them it was helpful? It's never too late. Graveside visits count.

Perhaps this doesn't strike you as a particularly meaty topic for a book of this nature, but I have a good reason for including it. Being grateful for the gifts we receive from others, gifts that fall into either the category of helpful suggestions or examples others set as they so peacefully lived their lives, can never be measured adequately. Perhaps that's because we so easily dismissed what our parents, and for sure our grandparents, told us or showed us because they were of different generations, thus they couldn't possibly relate to our world. What a silly idea. How ignorant too. Wisdom is wisdom and it's never outdated; it never loses value.

We all got many helpings of wisdom from our elders, and any single helping might well have made an important difference in some aspect of our life. Taking the time to review past encounters with these elders just may turn up a number of examples that are deserving of not only special recall, but a note of gratitude too. A literal note if they are still alive, or one shared in prayer if they have passed on.

Praising others for their contributions, large and small, to any area of one's life is exceedingly important I think. Why? Because knowing we have mattered to someone else is one of the triggers that makes everyone want to get up in the morning. We can only assume the same is true for everyone else too.

You have a job assignment: tell someone else how they helped you. Now.

Of course, many of those important contributions to our life were made by people who are now dead. Having to admit that we failed to talk to them before they died isn't something we need to feel shame over, because it's never too late to say thank you anyway. That's the good news. The really good news. Some reading this might not share my opinion that our loved ones, though bodily departed, are still present to us in spirit, but choosing to believe that has brought me hours of comfort. It has given me courage too.

When I think back on my life, I fear that one of the things I failed to mention to my mother was how proud I was of her for learning to drive a car at fifty-two. No one knew she was taking driving lessons. No one could have even guessed as much. The night she presented her license at the supper table became a celebration. I never asked my siblings if that act of hers affected them in any way, but I was changed by it. I learned, on the spot, that you were never too old to try something entirely knew. I also learned that you didn't need a cheering section either. She didn't have one. At least not until after the fact.

This is a gift I intend to pay homage to right now, in the same way as I'm suggesting you should. And how will I do this in the middle of this essay? Like this: I'll close my eyes. I will picture my mother behind the wheel of her little yellow Pinto. And I will say, "Thanks, Mom, for showing me what you were made of. It gave me courage to go to graduate school. It gave me courage to ride a motorcycle. It gave me courage to travel throughout Europe on business, even when I felt scared."

I so wish I had let her know how proud I was of her when she was still living. But I do think she knows now. That's how much I believe the Spirit world is as close as our thoughts.

Who would you like to show gratitude to before going any further? If he or she is still living, share here what you will do or say. If, like my mom, they have passed on, what is your plan? A prayer? A note at the graveside? A "talk" within a time of meditation? It doesn't matter what you choose. Just choose. The value will be registered anyway. It will bring value to your life as much as to her Spirit.

Dear _____:

The additional payoff from an act of gratitude, no matter how it is expressed, is that no one is untouched by it. No one. What is done for one is done for all. In the same way, what is done to one is done to all. There is no better reason for expressing kindness, gentleness, and generosity throughout our lives than this. We are either helping the universe through every action we take, or we are harming it. The choice, 24/7, is ours. Choose carefully.

When I think about others in my life that I want to thank, my grandmother comes to mind. I didn't have the wisdom or insight to tell her before she died how much I really loved her or learned from her, but I want her to know now. When I close my eyes I can still see her sitting low behind the wheel of the car, driving us to the park to ride the merry-go-round, a favorite treat every evening when we were in Logansport for our two-week summer vacation with her and my grandfather.

They dropped everything after supper to take us to the park and then to the Frozen Custard. We knew we were loved, even though I don't remember ever hearing those words. "Thank you both for making us feel special and loved."

And before turning this over to you and your notes of gratitude, I want to address one more person in my life. And it's my dad. We had a complicated relationship. He was often filled with rage. It came out at home. I fought back while my mom and my siblings looked on.

Our "dance" lasted well into adulthood. I did learn, at long last, that his anger was covering his fear. But what I learned from watching him through his rage and fear was that being afraid didn't have to immobilize you. He rose to the top at the bank anyway. He was elected the president of the banker's association in Indiana anyway. He ran Junior Achievement anyway. That meant that I, too, could succeed, even though I was afraid. It was a necessary lesson, or I would not have risen to the top of my organization. "Thank you, Daddy. I am really grateful for your strength in the face of fear."

———————

Your turn. Who are those people crying to be remembered? They are deserving of your homage. We all are deserving of your homage.

Thank you, thank you, thank you . . .

How does it feel to have taken care of this very important business of your life? I hope it feels good. What you have just done is offer wonderful gifts to those specific persons, along with the millions you will never know. But the tipping point is being "fed" with every show of gratitude, a gift to one and all.

———————

56

What's the Biggest Lesson of Your Life So Far?

Perhaps this question in a book of essays like these seems a bit lame. When it initially came to mind, I discarded it. It didn't feel meaty enough. Not soul-searching enough to measure up to the other essays. That's because I want to challenge you, and me too, to see who we really are beneath the surface that always *presents as fine,* and how we became the people we actually are today. Not surprisingly, further rumination clarified how important this question really is, and its necessity in a book like this. It might be the only worthy question to be asked and thoughtfully answered in this stage of life.

How often do any of us take stock of our lives? I'd venture to say not very often unless we were, or are, in therapy. Consider these questions, for example. Although they are rhetorical, please give them your attention. Make notes if that helps.

Where have you been, both physically and emotionally, at significant points throughout your lifetime?

Based on that information, where might you be headed next?

What cries out to you now as an adventure you'd like to explore, perhaps travel to an exotic land or college courses in poetry writing?

And last, what truly surprises you about your life so far?

Recalling our earlier lessons in search of the really big ones is one of the best indications I can think of for measuring what kind of person we have always sought to be. We need to evaluate our success. And if we didn't meet our expectations, what's the path we need to take to get where we want to be? Either now or next week.

It's not fair to ask you for your big lessons if I don't explore what mine are too. Not all my lessons have been positive, at least not initially. For instance, I learned the hard way what alcohol abuse could become. At thirteen, when I took that first drink, I had no idea how my world was going to change. Miraculously, I lived through many dangerous escapades.

Although I made lemonade from bushels and bushels of lemons, not everyone is so lucky. I learned how uncomfortable it was to lie to people who mattered to me, my parents for instance. I also learned what it felt like as an adult to talk about the thievery I committed as a child. I tried to laugh it off, but I was ashamed. I was afraid it would mar the reputation I had painstakingly developed as a writer of recovery books, work that required honesty. My fear was that my own recovery might be judged as questionable.

I learned what cheating with a friend's husband felt like. It was only fun for a very short while. I felt so ashamed that it destroyed our friendship, even though she never knew about the cheating. Alcohol had been the cause. That coupled with very poor judgment. I learned what my inability to trust men cost me emotionally. The list of tough lessons is a long one for me. But for every tough lesson, there was a good one, one that propelled me forward. And I came to believe that our lessons are always coupled that way. One tough lesson quickly followed by a good one.

I would have to say that the most profound, positive lesson I learned was that I had a Higher Power accompanying me down every bumpy road. This lesson carries over and infiltrates every fearful moment, reducing it to a manageable situation. Believing so wholeheartedly, as I do, that every lesson, all the tough ones as well as the easy ones, were bearing my name, gives a lightness to my step every day. Even though I had not accepted the comfort of that belief until I came into the 12-step rooms in the mid-seventies, like a soft blanket it had been wrapped around me anyway. How pleasing that knowledge is to me as an elder.

Perhaps the lesson that has been the most important is knowing that no one will ever cross my path who shouldn't. No one. On the contrary, every single person I meet, I have arranged to meet. I have written about this in earlier essays, but it had to be mentioned here again. You might not list this as one of your primary lessons, but that doesn't discount the truth of it in your life too. It's simply one of those basic truths for all humankind. We do not have to believe it for it to be true.

Every day, every moment, it pleases me to know I have been led to all the situations I have experienced. I was also led to my life partner Joe. We walk a compatible spiritual path, always supporting the journey we each are here to make. I have learned that love and acceptance are to be given away if we want to experience them ourselves. And I have learned that nothing ever has to be faced alone.

I have also learned the joy of studying. Surprisingly, every moment of graduate school pleased me and made me feel worthy. This is the biggest surprise of my life, actually. I had been convinced by my first husband that I'd never succeed, that I wasn't smart enough. But in 1979, the degree of Doctor of Philosophy from the University of Minnesota was granted to me anyway. To this day, I feel proud of that accomplishment.

And my work as a writer runs a very close second to my PhD. I had never expected to write a book, even though I had realized in graduate school that I loved writing more than anything I had ever done before. Loving writing and becoming a published writer don't always go hand in hand. Thirty books later, I'd have to say I'm tickled pink with my life. And it's my sincere hope that millions of readers have been helped by the work I love to do.

I know you have memories and lessons and successes and surprises too. How about beginning to share them here and now? The intention is to come face to face with your lifeline. Be cognizant of who you have actually been, warts and all. But you won't stop there. You will dwell on the memories in particular, coupled with their lessons. The successes deserve a special emphasis, particularly if they fostered blessings on others too. The section you might find the most fun are the surprises, most you won't have classified as that earlier. Hindsight allows us to see with such clarity. Most important of all, let this life review be fun. You deserve to enjoy this trip through your past. Now go and enjoy!

Memories: clear ones, sketchy ones, fun ones, difficult ones. Just remember, each one was necessary. Extremely necessary for you to be you.

Lessons: hard ones, easy ones, subtle ones, nearly forgotten ones.

Successes: ones that blessed others too, along with ones that were very quiet. Nothing is too small to mention, nor too big to mention. What you experienced had your name on it all along.

Surprises: the best part of looking back. Look at every decade, every one you have completed. Is there a conclusion you can draw from this list?

Take the time, before moving on, to record on tape a short history of all that is you, based on your collection of life events. Your family wants to really know you. This I can promise you. Do it now before it's too late.

57

Be a Mentor

*If I have the belief that I can do it, I shall surely acquire the
capacity to do it even if I may not have it at the beginning.*
— Mahatma Gandhi

The power inherent in believing that we can do something is
probably greater than any one of us estimates. And I'd guess
that hundreds of books have been published with the hope of
helping everyone increase their capacity to believe in themselves; believe in their prowess, their cleverness, their commitment to finishing something that was begun. Few of us stop to
consider very seriously, or at all, how valuable our willingness
to believe actually is.

When faced with a new challenge or when considering
whether to set a new goal, one unrelated to how you see yourself now, having the belief that the activity isn't beyond your
capacity to accomplish is crucial. When people don't believe in
themselves, they don't move beyond where they were as young
adults. We all know individuals who haven't grown. Men and
women who seem stuck in a mediocre past.

Let's count ourselves lucky to have been born with either
a naturally positive outlook, or to have been encouraged by
someone along the way to believe in ourselves, to believe in our
capacity to accomplish big things. It's a crucial quality to have if
one is seeking success.

Let's pay the same encouragement forward to some young
person in our circle of acquaintances. To really succeed takes

perseverance, the willingness to seek promotions, new jobs, and raises. Plus the willingness to follow the advice of your elders. You can encourage a young person in your life to dream big and accomplish those dreams.

It's my assumption that you have been rather successful and that you have more than just a slight belief in your capacity to try something new, or you probably wouldn't have purchased this book. It's probably not a book for everyone. But it is a book for the person who is still bent on living a full life, an exciting life, a life that continues to offer new adventures. My guess is that person also likes self-exploration, at least a small dose of it.

When you were young, did someone encourage you, mentor you, so to speak? Explain how that felt. What did it look like? How long was he or she in your life?

How might your life have looked if no one had encouraged you to go to the limit?

We can all see that our lives have been charmed in one way or another. I hope we can all see the value in helping to charm another young person's life. No one moves forward without taking others with them. Unfortunately, the reverse is just as true. Which side of the equation do you want to be on? I think I can guess.

In closing this essay, write an affirmation for yourself, an affirmation that joins you with a young person whom you can help. No one of us can do alone what every one of us can do in conjunction with another. The time is now. The place is here. Put one foot in front of the other and move forward. Help someone else find what you have found. And when the time is right, suggest they pay it forward too.

58

Lead by Example

Example is not the main thing in influencing others. It is the only thing.

—Albert Schweitzer

So many wonderful quotes are attributed to Albert Schweitzer. He lived as a great example to others of what a curious, committed, brilliant mind could accomplish. The following quote is also attributed to Schweitzer: "Constant kindness can accomplish much. As the sun makes ice melt, kindness causes misunderstanding, mistrust, and hostility to evaporate." It puts me in mind of Mother Teresa's quote about kindness that I love so much: "Be kind to everyone and start with the person standing next to you."

Striving to show up as a better person, in even the tiniest ways, makes a powerful contribution to the air we all breathe, to the mindset of anyone close by, to even the strangers we are certain live outside our reach. And yet, if we are to believe Schweitzer's quote, we are setting an example for others everywhere, every minute we are alive. Daunting idea, isn't it?

Frankly, I think it's an exciting idea that we are always serving as an example to others. Not only does it keep us on our toes, but it also gives us pause to remember all those individuals over the years who modeled good behavior for us. I mentioned this idea in an earlier essay and listed some of those key people in my life. I mention the idea again because praising others for the help they have shown us is such a kind thing to do. It's never too late to do so. Never too late.

This essay has two points, actually. The first one is to remind you that you are always making choices about how to behave in every situation. As a gauge for how good an example you are setting, consider whether your most common responses to people and situations would please your mother, if she were looking on. Or choose some other person you looked up to in your past. When we remember that our behavior is influencing others, that should give us reason to pause.

It's probably not every day that you think about the example you are setting. I'd have to admit that it's not on my mind very often either. However, whether we are conscious of it or not is irrelevant. We are being watched regardless. We have hundreds of chances every day to show our better side to anyone within earshot. I think it might be a good exercise for all of us to spend a few days watching others closely. What are you observing that you know you want to imitate? And the converse is to be noted too. Who do you not want to imitate?

Even though we are no longer in the prime of our lives, we still have plenty of time, no doubt many years, to practice good behavior, always discarding the behavior that serves as a poor example. Never forget, we are always being scrutinized, just as we still scrutinize others. That's a good thing, I think. Falling into the trap of thinking that what we are doing no longer matters to the world around us feeds the idea that we have become irrelevant. Not so. Never will it be so.

In order to maximize the full benefit of this essay, I think we (I'm including myself in this investigation) need to make a list of all those people who come quickly to mind whose behavior has been a great example to us as we developed into the persons we are today. Even though we were also, unfortunately, occasionally influenced by behavior that wasn't stellar, we need not take stock of that now. The more we focus on good behavior from both the past and the present, the more likely we will be to model good behavior for others.

To demonstrate my purpose here, I'll go first. You can then model yourself after me.

A few people I looked up to in my early formative years:

My Grandmother Kirkpatrick. She was always kind and never argued with anyone, and she never talked about people in a negative way.

Bob Priest, my sixth grade teacher. Mr. Priest never had favorites in our classroom. He was kind, yet strict. And he trusted us enough to bring all of us to his cabin on the Wabash River on the last day of school.

Don Rivers, my boss at Loeb's when I was in high school. I did mention him before, but he's worth a second mention. He respected my ability to be good in sales. He made me feel like I mattered to the success of our clothing department, and he put me in charge of some key assignments. That's what really mattered.

Before I move on to those people who influenced me in the next stage of my life, please look at your own formative years. You may not recall many at first; however, this isn't a race to be done. It's far more important to take the time necessary to look back. Who was in your circle and stood out for you?

Those who come to mind are . . .

I married while still in Purdue and my life was so focused on partying, before and after Bill and I married, that I allowed very few people to influence me in a positive way. I was far more focused on following in the footsteps of people who were walking on the edge. One person does come to mind, however. I mentioned him in essay 37, but giving him another high five here is important. What he did for me stuck with me all through graduate school.

Ray Firnstahl was his name. He was creative, experimental in the classroom, and always in favor of stretching the limits the school district put on us. He wasn't afraid of being challenged where the future of the children under his care was concerned. He was principled in every way. His mindset was worthy of imitation.

Nobody else stands out until I entered graduate school following my divorce from Bill. And then the flood gates open. Men and women galore served as great examples of honesty, integrity, perseverance, and love. And since that time there have been even more individuals who stand out. They are almost too numerous to list, but I think it's important for me to write their names in this public place, so I will never forget who they were.

Individuals who mattered, really mattered to who I have become because of the example they set get mentioned here. It wasn't what they told me, but what they showed me through their lives that really mattered:

Mulford Sibley, Roger Buffalohead, Toyce Kyle, my mother, Thelma Elliott, Harry Swift, Pat Butler.

There are many more, but my point has been made. Those people who influenced us to become who we have become are worthy of our thanks and our public acknowledgement. Because of them, and many more, I have become a woman that others may choose to imitate in some way. Hopefully my example, at least in this last half of my life, has been good.

Now it's your turn. You can do this exercise however and wherever you choose to do it. My point is only this: do it! It will be good for you. We are composites of all who went before us and we will influence all who look to us. There is still time remaining to become more of who we really want to be.

In closing this essay, let me simply say bravo for a memory well served. We are part and parcel of all we have seen, all we have heard, all we have longed for. If we do nothing more of import in our remaining years, we can feel satisfied that, indeed, we have done enough. But people like us are always looking for the next challenge to survive. Go with confidence that your past has fully prepared you for anything that the present will ever toss toward you. Trust me. I know you because I know me.

59

What Makes You Come Alive?

Don't ask what the world needs. Ask what makes you come alive and go do it. Because what the world needs is people who have come alive.

—Howard Thurman

Have you ever given any consideration to what really rings your chime at this stage of life? Maybe it's similar to what really got your attention when you were much younger. For instance, I still love writing, obviously. This is my thirtieth book. I first knew that I loved to write as a child. And then in graduate school, I knew it at a deeper level. To have made a living as a writer has been such a blessing, and I can foresee writing at least another five or six, or even ten, books. As I said in an earlier essay, I can imagine following in Frida Kahlo's footsteps, writing even on my deathbed. That idea doesn't seem an odd one to me at all.

What were you doing for the sheer joy of it when you were entering the workforce? Perhaps you were as lucky as me and were able to do the very thing you loved more than any other activity, the very thing that made you come alive, as Thurman put it. And get paid for it. But if that wasn't the case, and more than likely it wasn't, there was something that called to you outside work. There always is something that calls to us. But often, we ignore those calls, feeling like there's no time for them. Making a living is all we have time for.

That was then. This is now. Doing something fun is calling to you. Perhaps a mentoring program where you work with young people to help them find direction. I have met a handful of people who are retired from their profession who are involved in just such a program and they love it. Interestingly, two of them never had children. Maybe it's a part-time job for extra money that calls to you, and you love it because you are with the public. I have a neighbor who is a greeter at Walgreens. She says she loves it. It gets her out of the house and with people a few hours daily.

Tutoring is an interest of many. In a much earlier period of my life, I taught second and third grade and I loved it. Helping children learn, seeing their eyes light up when they understand a new concept, is deeply rewarding. And best of all, you know you are responsible for lighting a fire in this child, one that can never be entirely extinguished. Coming back to this in a later stage of life calls to me. My main concern presently is time. I'm still working too much to allow for many other activities. I keep thinking, *When I get old* . . . and then I remember I am seventy-five. When am I old enough?

Has anything begun to call to you yet? Perhaps making a list of what you see others doing will help your mind open up to new and unexpected ideas. It's worth a try. Begin by interviewing your own friends about what they would like to explore, or maybe have already explored, as they have more time on their hands. One of my women friends volunteers as a guardian *ad litem* in the court system. She finds representing young children very rewarding.

Like me, she too was a school teacher. Perhaps my service as a teacher is too long ago to make that a good activity for me, but I do worry about children in families where drugs and alcohol are taking a toll. Being a support person for them would make sense to me since my own past was riddled with alcoholism and drug abuse. Fortunately, I didn't bring children into my world then.

I love Thurman's quote because it makes me smile. Thinking about people who are truly alive is a treat. We notice them so easily. Something about them simply appears different from so many others. They may not always be smiling, but they seem to have an inner sizzle that grabs your attention. When you notice people over the next week or two who seem really happy, dare to ask them what makes them so happy. Additionally, ask what one thing makes them happiest of all?

As I'm thinking about this essay, perhaps it's unreasonable to expect you to know what it is that makes you want to hop out of bed now if you aren't working a regular job anymore. I just had the realization that if I were reading this in another author's book, how would I respond? It makes sense to me to tell you what I do that makes me sizzle in the morning. Because I do get up anticipating a great day, even though I'm not as retired as many of you are who are reading this.

I have my coffee, of course. That's a must. I engage in a conference call with a group of women for a spirituality discussion based on a reading from a book. We do this at 7:10 central standard time, every morning. Next I check my email, which is also a must. Because I am still working, I stay on top of emails because I receive requests for workshops, lectures, dinner talks, etc., and I want to be responsive immediately. Next I check in with the morning news.

Most importantly of all, my husband and I read from *A Course in Miracles* every morning, which helps each of us to center ourselves spiritually and be on the same page. This has been a crucial addition to our marriage. My last prep for the day is a walk, during which I pray for all my family and friends, for their peace and wellbeing, for their health and happiness. And if any one person is having a tough struggle, he or she gets an extra dose of prayer.

Now I'm ready for whatever is needed from me for the day. Generally I spend a number of hours doing exactly what I am doing right now: writing. And the time flies. I feel a sense of satisfaction, and I know that keeping this as one of my go-to activities for the rest of my life will ensure that I feel complete. What could be better? What indeed?

Why don't you do the exercise I just did so you can assess how your life actually looks, now, on a normal day? See what you learn from doing that. Try to gather some information about what brings you joy right now. Kind of look over your own shoulder to see what's really peeking out. And make a list of those things. Before you forget them:

My joys.

My longings.

My plan for tomorrow.

And the next day.

I will be content if . . .

Share your thoughts with others who may be searching too. We all need a guide for doing some new thing that has called to us. We all need a friend to walk through these new times with. If you don't already have one, picture the kind of friend you want so that she or he can find you.

60

Age Aside

Age aside, it's never too late to make a new ending.

—Phil Burgess, PhD

I love this quote. It actually comes from a personal friend of nearly sixty years. We both graduated from high school in 1957 in Indiana. He wrote a meaty book, also about this latter stage of life, titled *Reboot! What to Do When Your Career Is Over but Your Life Isn't.* His premise, like mine, is that we aren't done, even if at first it appears that way. We always have more to offer. Always. And the community around us deserves to benefit from our continuing vitality. Our lives remain quite purposeful, even though what we had considered our primary purpose for the many years of our career has come to an end.

Actually, I have met very few people approaching retirement or even already in retirement who say they want to simply sit down and read books. Or play golf. Or learn to play bridge. It's certainly okay if that's what a person prefers, and I think everyone should take at least a brief timeout before diving into an activity of any kind, just to recharge the inner core.

But withdrawing from the human community, for more than a couple months following that big retirement party, begins to extinguish the spirit within. And that's never to our benefit. No matter how tired we may be from a demanding career, letting the spirit flicker and die eventually steals our peace of mind, that very thing we sought more of, throughout our journey here.

I am obviously not in the retired mode yet, or you wouldn't be reading this book. But I am moving in that direction, which is what pulled me to write this book. Now. It's been on my mind for some time. And the haunting question for me, even though it's not for many of the people in my circle of friends and acquaintances, is who will I be when I am not the me who is sitting here at the computer still working?

As I have said in earlier essays, I'm pretty certain that writing will always call to me in some form. My passion for it simply burns too bright for it to quietly die. And that comforts me. What's going to call to you? I promise that something will if you allow yourself to dream. And are you prepared to follow the thread wherever it leads you? It could lead you to a faraway land, perhaps. Or into a new relationship, even a new business partnership, or perhaps having a hobby that actually begins to pay dividends. An experience you had never imagined would occur.

Try playing a little game with yourself. First, just close your eyes and empty your mind. After a few minutes, let your mind wander. Let it go wherever it wants. When it lights on something that pulls it in, imagine yourself being an actual part of the picture you see. Don't edit your thoughts. Let them be as wild as they want to be. That may be the clue you need to discover where your next stage of living will take you.

Knowing that nothing is really off limits as long as it's legal leaves many choices—hundreds, in reality. I think the only thing we should consider is whether or not what we choose to do will benefit others. That leaves our next stage wide open doesn't it? Perhaps you think that I'm placing a limit on you by saying it should be of benefit to others. It's been my experience, particularly with the thousands of people I have worked with over the years in hundreds of workshops, that when the choices we make hurt others, they hurt us even more. So choose with an open heart among all the myriad ideas that spring into your mind.

If you still have no idea how you want to spend your time when you have more of it on your hands, reading the book *What Color Is Your Parachute? for Retirement, Second Edition: Planning a Prosperous, Healthy, and Happy Future* by John E. Nelson and Richard N. Bolles may send you down a perfect path.

I remember reading the original *What Color Is Your Parachute?* book by Bolles following completion of my PhD in 1979. I knew writing was my passion, but I also knew I might have to settle for something else. It helped to confirm where my interests were. And more importantly, where they were not. My first job was in publishing, and it also eventually led to an opportunity to write my first book. The rest is history, as they say.

The point I'm trying to make is that we still have so much to offer others and for many years to come. Being stymied about our future can lead to doing too little for too long, which can lead to losing hope that we will ever feel okay. We need to lead a meaningful life. At every age. It's as simple as that. Nothing less than that will satisfy us, and the very fact of our continuing existence demands it.

I well remember reading the book *Illusions* by Richard Bach nearly forty years ago. I was trying to get through a very dark period of my life. After completing the book, I turned it over to read the back cover copy. *Bingo!* To paraphrase, it said, "If you are reading this back page now, you have yet to fulfill your purpose." I was thrilled. I felt saved. It gave me exactly the boost I needed to believe that I would be okay. I did have a purpose, a fact that I had never believed before.

We must remember and celebrate that we bring all the meaning our lives will ever know to everything we see, to everything we do. Having the power to determine the meaning in and of itself increases the level of passion we will feel around whatever we choose to do. And the choices are as many and as varied as one can imagine. Bolles's book can help narrow down the choices because it offers so many ways to evaluate them. But his book isn't the only one that might help. Sticking with the book you are currently holding, doing all the exercises that I have suggested, will definitely point you in the right direction for stage four, perhaps the best stage of all. So some of us think.

The really good news, if you haven't discovered it yet, is that your life is about to become more fun and more interesting than you could ever have imagined. Now, because nothing is really holding you back, you can dream big and do big things. No one can stop you. No one but your critical ego, and you can choose to ignore him. In fact, the ego has never and will never want you to succeed. It never really did. Fortunately, you always had those two voices in your mind, the one that encouraged you, and the other one. Every time you listened to the wrong voice, you paid for it.

You and I are free now. No longer need we fear (if we ever did) someone looking over our shoulder and reprimanding us. How we spend the hours of every day, whether in the company of others or alone, whether enjoying a hobby or working part time, we need do nothing but be attentive and kind to the others whom we encounter. It's as simple as that. And if push comes to shove, we don't even have to be kind. Attentiveness is always a gift though. Rapt attention is the kindest of all gifts. Our unkindnesses, however, will come back to bite us. Bite us hard. Let's avoid that. And send good ions into the atmosphere around us. That's the best kind of work for any age. And this is an idea you can take to the bank!

Let's play a while. What's the wildest but still fun, safe thing you can imagine doing, now that you have all this new freedom?

What's the upside of the above activity?

Is there a downside?

Make a list of all the benefits that accrue from this choice.

Why did this activity choose you?

What can you imagine as the biggest payoff from this choice?

Who comes quickly to mind as the beneficiaries of this choice?

Before ending this essay, what help have the brief exercises been?

Do you feel a sense of direction emerging?

What direction are you now pointed in?

Sit with this choice for a few days and then, not before, begin exploring the particulars of how this choice might play out in your life.

What about it feels good?

When you feel ready, go for it. Then check back with this essay and report how you feel.

Do you think this has been a good choice for you?

And if you have discovered that's it's not so good, no harm has been done.

Beginning the process again will be even more fun. I promise.

Ready, set, go!

61

Say What You Need to Say

What do you want to say to a close friend or family member but haven't been able to say? In 12-step recovery rooms, where I have spent the last forty years, we focus on making amends to those individuals we harmed in some way during our using days, unless the amend would harm that person all over again. I know that making amends for my many transgressions freed me from the shame and guilt that dogged my steps. Not everyone understood the process. I'm not sure everyone believed my behavior was actually going to change. My father believed my alcoholism was what had kindled my insistence that I was always right whenever we argued. I'm sure that contributed to it. So did *his* insistence that *he* was always right. That contributed even more.

When I began my spiritual journey in 1974, with the aid of the 12 steps, I lost my taste for conflict. It actually had always scared me, even when I was a willing participant, a fear that was given birth to while I was still a child in a household where alcohol and arguments were prevalent, a household where I suffered perpetual stomachaches. But now I didn't want to participate in a conflict at all. What freedom that offered.

And with the aid of the spiritual program I was committed to, my behavior did change, little by little, one day at a time. I had not simply chosen to drink no more and abstain from chemicals of every kind. I had also decided to behave in a far quieter, consistently more loving way. It felt good. I was relieved of much of the anxiety that had haunted me for years. I wish I could say that all my anxiety was gone. Alas, that was not the case, but its lessening was very healing. And it gave me hope.

Many of you reading this book may not have been exposed to any of my other books, or to any 12-step group either. But it's my guess that most of you would trade conflict for peaceful experiences in a flash. And throughout this book, I have tried to help you find ways to enhance your journey, fostering greater peace, in this latter stage of life. And giving to others what we would like to experience from them is life altering, for them and for us. And it instills an eagerness for each day's passage because of the myriad renewed opportunities to pay forward a bit of kindness.

Remember the book *All I Really Need to Know I Learned in Kindergarten,* written by Robert Fulghum? The wisdom within that book, within the idea itself, if lived, would change the universe. Using the simple wisdom of childhood as your guide, you can quickly assess what words you need to share with others, whether they are amends or words of praise. Life is so much simpler than we make it. Let's begin, now, to simplify. But let's clean up the past, any part of it that needs to be made right, before we embark on this journey of simplification.

When I look over my life, who are the key people who have always mattered to me? Listing all of them in my journal, and giving a few moments of meditation to each one, will jar my memory if there is something I need to address with them. Here goes.

It's my guess that you might have had many pleasant recollections, among whatever else came to your mind. What fun those are. And among those recollections, something will inspire you, perhaps, to pursue it in this final, major stage of life. As I live more into it, day by day, I am greeting each day a bit more lightheartedly. At seventy-five, the heavy lifting is over. All done. Whew! And the best may yet to be come. I do believe, absolutely, that if I think the best is yet to come, what comes next will be the best, the very best. We get what we "order." That's a promise.

Let's return to that list of people who have mattered to you. Do you see a pattern in the kind of clean-up you may need to do? It's not surprising if that's the case. And that's fortuitous. It means that the behavior we still have time to change falls into easily managed categories. I know that if I were doing the exercise I've suggested that you do, I'd need to address my inclination to judge others. Seldom do I do it audibly, so it's not likely I have to make a formal apology. But I do need to ask for help from my Higher Power to make the shift in perception that is called for.

One significant feature of my spiritual path that I've referred to in other essays is *A Course in Miracles.* It offers easy principles that lead to the change in my behavior that is so appealing; in fact, the course has become necessary if I want to live peacefully. And I do.

It's your turn. What are those few behaviors you need to put a halt to now?

And now that you know what they are, what behavior will you substitute?

Let's return to the fun parts of growing older. And I do mean fun parts. We don't have to perform for anybody. We can get up when we want to, get dressed when we want to, eat what we want to, fat free or not. I remember suggesting to my mom when she was my current age that she may want to forego a particular food because it was so fattening. She put me straight in no uncertain terms. With firmness she said, "At my age, I will eat whatever I damn well please!"

I have followed in her footsteps often, and I, too, would say the very same thing now if I had a daughter who said that to me. Maybe that's one of the good reasons for not having had children, although I never thought about it at the time of all the failed pregnancies.

Aging frees us to do whatever we want, really. I want you to go there now. I want you to dream big. I want you to expand your consciousness. Whether you do all that you imagine doing or not is not the point. What comes to mind? Write it down. Now.

Sit back now and breathe deeply. The future is yours to make. Tread lightly but steadily forward. There are days and years awaiting your presence. You will be at peace. At peace. Then and now.

———————————

62

Your Timeline

There have been no mistakes in how one's life has unfolded. This is a spiritual truth. This is a truth that had to grow on me. I was introduced to it when I came into the 12-step rooms in 1974, but I resisted it at first. In particular, I resisted the assurance with which the idea was pushed at me. It seemed just too convenient. I had no doubt heard the idea prior to 1974, but had never given it much credence. It was one of those ideas that seemed easy to dismiss. And now, some forty years later, I consider it one of the most treasured of all the truths l live by. It's curious, I think, that many ideas I treasured prior to recovery no longer even rank a place in my memory bank. They didn't survive the test of time. And the ones I considered not particularly important in my early recovering days are honored by me now.

I very much like this particular spiritual truth because of the comfort it has provided in regard to some of the less pleasant experiences I've encountered in my seventy-five years on the planet. I've mentioned a number of these already, so I don't need to repeat a lot of that detail again. But I am thrilled to claim this truth as one of the basic foundations of my life. I think we all need, in fact we always needed, a set of beliefs we could rely on to support us. Without them, we are left floundering, trying to make sense of lives that don't, on the surface, always appear rational.

This essay, you might begin to note, is a bit different. I'm changing the pace for purposes of interest, I hope. I'm not sure if you have ever been asked to create a timeline before.

Some of you may not know what I mean, in fact. But a timeline is a linear line either across the page or up and down the side of a page, and on the line, memorable experiences, both good ones and bad ones, are listed at their approximate year of occurrence.

For instance, my timeline would include falling down two flights of steps onto a concrete floor into our basement when I was two years old. I refused to be held or comforted by my older sister and my mother, who had both run down the steps to hold me. I wouldn't let them pick me up. I refused to even cry, I have been told.

The timeline would also include an emergency appendectomy at age seven. The first time I was sexually molested at age ten. My first drink at thirteen would be noted at its proper point on the line, as well as my first consensual sexual encounter at seventeen. Getting secretly married at twenty, an unfortunate decision, would show up on the line too. And this is just the beginning.

The timeline will best be tackled in a journal and will consume your attention for a few hours. Possibly it will be done a bit every day for a few days. Don't be concerned about time. It's the history that's remembered that is important. You won't have total recall of your life. But I think you will see a pattern emerging. I've suggested this task to many people in workshops, and there has always been a pattern. Oftentimes, one that amazed the participants.

Once the specific experiences have been recalled and put on paper, some of you will have a hundred or more. I suggest that quiet reflection be given to each recollection. This is your life, after all. Your unique, extremely special life, a life that has intersected with hundreds, perhaps thousands of people in a very preordained way. This is the juicy part of the essay. Allowing yourself the time to fully recall, and in full detail, the experiences from your life, is a gift you deserve. Now. What a delicious undertaking.

No one knows you like you do. Not even a therapist you may have seen for years. Not a life partner either. We are all good at making up stories about our loved ones, what we think their many experiences said about them. But no one has lived in our minds. You, and only you, get to know the whole of you. No one but you can fill in all the blanks, so to speak.

Perhaps you are wondering why I'm suggesting you do this? The answer is simple. There is no time like now to celebrate the life you have presented to the world. Every moment we breathe brings us closer to the last breath we will take, so celebrating the gifts we have given and received in our time on this planet is an experience you deserve. Every single one of your experiences added another thread that was woven into the tapestry that is you. And every tapestry, still being created by every one of us, all seven billion and counting, keeps adding to the brilliance of the universe we share.

You need to revisit every event for what it was in its moment, but even more, for how it contributed to making you the man or woman you are today, sixty or seventy years later. The man or woman who is now on the threshold of saying, "It's time to slow down and appreciate the smaller, quieter moments in life." I know, even though I am still at my desk, on my computer, sending these suggestions out to you, that my time to slow down is calling to me.

The timeline was not meant to be busywork. Remember as youngsters in school when the teachers would hand out worksheets that were simply busywork to keep us quiet and engaged so the teacher could work with another reading group, perhaps? This timeline was not one of those assignments. And if you approached it right, it did keep you interested while others around you went about their own lives. Never has anyone been as interesting to us as ourselves. I think we can bank that statement.

But celebrating the fullness of every event of your life, paying it the homage it deserves, is one of the greatest of all pleasures in our advancing years. We lived each moment. We deserved each moment. Let's remember each moment. Let's honor each moment. The universe around us would not be what it is without each and every single experience that all seven billion of us have had. What an awesome truth that is. How extremely important it makes absolutely every tiny detail of every life that has ever been lived.

In closing this essay, I want to say I hope you save this timeline for all the years that remain. I hope you continue adding to it. And most of all, I hope you share it with someone you love very much. Let him or her know you in a deeper way. The most intimate way, in fact. And then look at each decade and pick the three things that are most important to you now, but that happened in that decade.

When you have that list of thirty or forty experiences, make a summary statement about each decade. Put these summary statements together and review your life. Are you pleased? I hope so. I promise, you did what you came to do. You met who you had planned to meet. You effected who you needed to effect. You learned what you came to learn. And you will continue to do exactly this until that last breath is taken. Your mission is ongoing. Honor what remains.

63

Life's "Accidents"

Since most of you reading this book are either already in or are about to enter the final quarter of your life, you may have decided that change, whether living it or doing it or causing it, isn't all that important anymore. *Whatever will be will be.* There's nothing wrong with looking at your life from that perspective; however, being more proactive can guarantee a series of choice experiences. And who wouldn't rather live more peacefully with our loved ones? Who among us wouldn't prefer less anxiety when in the company of strangers? And is there any one of us who really wants to cultivate more chaos to wade through? I think the answer to all of these questions is obvious. Stillness is simply inviting. It's contagious, healing, and inspired. It's the gold ring we reach for when riding a carousel.

Every one of us has lived through thousands of changes on our way to this book. And every single change, absolutely every one of them, made by you and, likewise, made by me, was necessary for us to get to *this point* of our intersection. That idea gives me goose bumps. Honest to God goose bumps that stand out on my arms. There are no accidents. Absolutely none. None at all.

As a fun exercise, take a short break here and think about some of the "accidents" that stand out prominently in your mind. Perhaps the ones that seemed so counter to the direction you thought you were going in. Make that list in your journal now.

What were your unexpected experiences, labeled by some as "accidents"?

Do you detect any pattern to these changes? If not at first glance, look again more slowly.

Which changes opened doors to experiences you'd never have imagined happening to you?

What changes did you hate at first, only to eventually develop a bonding attachment to them?

Which change, or two, has had the most lasting effect on you?

Let's go back to the bigger picture again. Many of us probably wanted to "incite" or dispel more than one change at some point in our life. I'm well aware of my attempt to change my first husband's mind about leaving me. It wasn't because of my undying love. On the contrary, it was because of my shame over being left for another woman. Nothing I said or did could dissuade him, however. The pain at that time felt unbearable. And it was solely because I felt embarrassed. None of my friends had been left by their husbands. I was grateful to be able to drown my sorrows in alcohol, never realizing that it, too, was very gradually pushing me into a rich, very rewarding life; one I could never have imagined for myself, one that included believing in a Source greater than myself.

What I couldn't see through the tears then were the many doors that were opening to a new, exciting life, one that included 12-step recovery, earning a PhD, and becoming the author of thirty books (with no end in sight). The silver lining was blinding, indeed. What I want to stress is that your life was also wrapped in a cloak that had a silver lining, a cloak you may have paid little heed to. Now is the time to pay homage, however. *Now.*

With fresh eyes I look around. Here is what I see . . .

And what makes me happiest is . . .

And now, on to the better world that I choose to see and then live.

Living in the Moment with Rapt Attention

Make every task you undertake, or person you encounter, your universe for the moment. Rapt attention, as I mentioned in an earlier essay, surpasses in value every other character trait we may possess. The decision to honor our fellow travelers with devoted attention, in regard to their every word, their loud as well as their quiet behavior, their very presence in our lives regardless of what the expression is, is a gift beyond measure. This idea may feel suffocating when first considered. However, it offers anyone who embraces it freedom at a very deep level. No other decision about life's journey and our responses to anyone we will ever encounter on our journey ever needs to be made. *Not ever.*

I'm of course not sure how this suggestion for how to see your life registers with you. Giving your rapt attention to the people around you sounds extreme. I know. But I have grown extremely fond of the idea. It has reduced the stress in my life immeasurably. For decades, my mind was consumed with thoughts, things, responses, judgments, opinions, and negativities of every persuasion that I attached to whomever or whatever was *even possibly* out there. The busyness of my mind was debilitating and exhausting. Being told I didn't need to live that way anymore was suspect. Being attentive to *this moment's universe* seemed like an impossible and rather uninteresting way to live. My mind was *out there*, mixing it up with whoever I conjured up, no matter what was right here in front of me.

And then one day, as the result of studying *A Course in Mir-*

acles, I woke up to the truth that *there is no out there.* I was gob-smacked. Never was there an out there, the course taught. What we see out there is what we have projected from our own mind. Never more. Never less. Giving my rapt attention to only what is right here and now before me, no matter how inconsequential it may seem to be, is a gift sent from God. And I mean that literally.

Some of you have no doubt lived in the moment for years. Some spiritual philosophies teach this. I tip my hat to you. Constant, vigilant practice was necessary for me to fully embrace that nothing but *now* existed and then learn how to live only in the now. I still stumble occasionally. Some days many times, but the payoff each time I do embrace the present moment is sweet. It leaves a pleasant taste in my mouth. It feels like a comforter around my shoulders on a cool evening. It relieves me of even a hint of anxiety. I trust that the God of my understanding is paying me a visit within every moment of my life, and I'll miss his call if my mind is on the past or guessing about some future event. Or more than likely, passing judgment on the people in my past or projected future.

Giving up our reliance on the past to define the present is a must if we ever want to experience the peace that we are promised when we stay saddled in the comfort of now. I have decided that I am too old to relish conflict. In a very unhealthy way, I used to thrive on it. It frightened me, but it also made me feel alive. Now it scares me. There is only one way to avoid being frightened. I must step into this moment and cherish it. This is an assignment I can happily accept.

I have made a case for living here and now. I hope you can see that. Now it's your turn to evaluate your progress with this idea. And if you haven't mastered the way to do it, you are like most of the human race. We grow into older age still fumbling in the past or living in dread of some future task assigned to us. Being told that we don't have to live like this anymore may seem a bit hard to comprehend and then believe. But it's true. I promise that it's true. All that will convince you, however, is the results of practicing how to focus on what presents itself on your path, minute by minute. There are no shortcuts. Simply do it. And be gentle with yourself each time you fall into the ditch of an old habit.

Let's note, minute by minute, what's in our range of attention right now. If this seems laborious, just trust me, it will jar you from your past. I'll demonstrate what I'm asking you to do.

For me right now are the following:

Shoulder tension; the sound of a fan behind me; the tapping of my nails on the keyboard; relief at being inside the house rather than walking in the hot sun; the words that are flowing onto this page; the wellbeing I feel doing this work; the dog sitting in the shade of the tree next door; the quietness of my life in this moment; the certainty that God is here, now; the awareness that nothing will disturb me, ever, unless I let it; the stack of mail to be addressed; my iPad next to me; my always present bottle of water; my file boxes holding copies of workshop outlines, expenses, etc.; framed art on the walls; and pictures of family and friends on bookshelves. My mind is simply open to whatever my muse offers me, which I tap out on the keys.

I am completely at peace. I know I'm being cradled by the God of my understanding. And I know no decision or action or even any tiny thought needs to be determined by me. God and I will create it together.

Now I'd like for you to do this exercise. If you find yourself slipping into the past while trying to live in the moment, don't be concerned. Let that slide right by.

At this moment . . .

In order to strengthen your commitment to experiencing life as simply one encounter of *now* after another, practice this exercise daily for at least twenty-one days. Doing this exercise multiple times a day will be helpful. When we are told that something this simple can have a profound impact on our life and our daily wellbeing, wouldn't we be foolish not to practice it? I think so. You will too, once you see the change in the tenor of your life. My guess is that you will be telling others soon after to try it too. Carry on . . .

———————

65

You Can't Change Others, So Change Yourself

He who has so little knowledge of human nature as to seek happiness by changing anything but his own disposition will waste his life in fruitless efforts.

—Samuel Johnson

I feel fortunate to have embraced the principle that Samuel Johnson espouses in the above quote many decades ago. Had I not been introduced to a 12-step recovery program in my thirties, I may not have stumbled on it in such a profound way. My life had always been about trying to change others, *any others*, to safeguard my journey. But from my first day in "the rooms," I caught a glimmering from these kind strangers that my belief was folly. Complete folly. At the very least.

Fortunately I stuck around and began to soak up what these wise men and women had to say, because I had few other options. I either had to change my life and opt for sobriety, or continue tripping down dark alleys where booze was cheap and people were cheaper, finally ending at the door marked "death." Not everybody following the path I was on is lucky enough to get off. For some it's just too late. Way too late. I went to the wakes for more than a few of them.

Part of my journey into alcoholism was because I was shattered by my fear of abandonment by others, even though the full force of what I anticipated seldom happened. For it to happen even once was enough, however. From then on I watched like a hawk every man who paid attention to me and drowned my fears, night after night, in a bottle of Jack Daniel's.

As a teenager, I had never considered where I wanted to go in life. My mother told me many years ago that when I was small, I said I wasn't going to have babies. I wanted to be "a working lady." I've thought about that thousands of times over the years. As the saying goes, "Out of the mouths of babes . . ." I never gave birth. And I did work. More specifically, however, I hung my future on whomever seemed to want me around.

I graduated from Purdue University in 1962 with a degree in elementary education, a minor in psychology, and a philandering husband who moved us to Minneapolis, Minnesota, where he, rather haphazardly, pursued a graduate degree and other women while I taught school. As happens all too often in ill-conceived marriages, ours ended after twelve recklessly alcoholic years because of another woman. One of many other women. And my journey into unbridled, unabridged alcoholism was born.

I have told my story many times in meetings and within the pages of numerous books, and the one certainty I have come to accept is that the trajectory of my life was intentional, even divine, I'd say, from the moment of conception. I doubt not that every experience I ever had was necessary to the tapestry I was born to weave. I find that idea extremely comforting. From my perspective, little time, if any, needs to be spent trying to analyze why my life took the twists and turns it did. I know, without a shadow of a doubt, that I needed to meet whom I met. I needed to learn what I learned. And I taught whomever crossed my path just as they were teaching me.

There is certainly no reason to expect an unplanned-for interruption in the flow of my life now. Whatever direction I am nudged to follow in what I consider to be my last quarter will be as perfect as my first seventy-five years. I will follow any nudge wherever it leads me, knowing that I am fulfilling the perfect plan for me. And my joy with the specifics is my choice. And only my choice.

How fortunate I feel that this perfect plan has embedded in me many wise and worthy concepts, like the quote by Samuel Johnson, an idea that has allowed me, actually encouraged me, to create my own happiness in the blink of an eye. The very idea that I could do such a thing seemed impossible while I was wandering along the scarred path of my life, drinking in bars where I knew no one, wandering into parties that seemed to have no exit. But all the while I was being watched over. I didn't have to know this for it to be true. *And wherever you were, or are, this is your truth too.*

Growing old with the wisdom of many of my elders, those I know or knew in the flesh, and those I just read about in the many volumes I studied while earning my PhD, gave me a frame of reference to begin hanging my tapestry on. My tapestry, though not yet complete, comforts me. I know that every thread contributed exactly what I needed at the time.

What I didn't understand, for much of my life, however, was that I was *not a victim. Not ever,* even though I chose to think so on many occasions. Being able to believe and then celebrate that *nothing was ever done to me* is life-changing. It's also attitude changing. Like Johnson so wisely told us, the choice to be happy or not falls to us. Abraham Lincoln concurred. He has been quoted as saying, "You are as happy as you make up your mind to be." In other words, it's our responsibility to be happy, to be productive, to be courageous—no one else's. And when we absorb this idea fully, as no doubt most of you have, it assures us that our purpose was always carefully charted, and protected, while we were being prepared for whatever was next on the great agenda of our lives.

And now here we are in 2015, awaiting the future while squeezing every breath of life from the present. Hopefully. The purposeful future. We all have one. I know this absolutely. I know you know it too at some level. Do we need to plan it? I think not. Not in detail anyway. What's more important, I think, is to trust in the inspiration that calls us forward when we get ourselves out of the way.

Getting ourselves out of the way is the challenge for most of us. And how is this done? Those of you who are regularly meditating have already mastered this. Those who haven't yet explored this glorious activity are in for a treat. Our inspiration waits for us there. It's patient. It's quiet. It's specific. And like one's inner guide who has always been with us, the message he or she has for us is ours alone. Our purposeful future won't "get away."

––––––––––––––––––

Change of pace . . .

Let's play with this idea for a few minutes. Just for fun. Close your eyes. Empty your mind. Settle into your chair. Breathe deeply. Again and again. I know reading this and trying to do what I'm suggesting seems counterproductive, but read first and then set all of this aside. Take at least ten minutes to allow yourself to really quiet your mind. And then the inner action will begin. It may seem at first that everything in your mind is all jumbled up. Running from one topic into another. It is, in fact, but that's part of the process. Don't be discouraged, and don't give up before the miracle.

If you are open to some guidance about the next phase of the journey, if you have requested this guidance, it will come. It may not seem at first that what comes to mind was meant for you. But stay quiet. Keep asking for help. That which is wearing your name will come forth. Remember, the pact was made eons ago. But it was made nonetheless. Even if it doesn't seem like a choice you would have made, remember, two souls were choosing. You were one of them. Your teacher was the other. And lest you think that we are done learning in this latter stage of living, think again. Some of our best lessons lie ahead, and that's because we have more time and less stress in our lives.

And if you keep meditating and nothing very contextual comes to mind, consider that its own special gift. When you are needed, you will be called. In the meantime, what are some activities that appeal to you? Feel free to try one or all of them. Just know without a doubt that since you are still alive, you have a purpose to fulfill. It will find you.

No go out for ice cream and relax.

———————————

66

Is Real Peace Ever an Actuality?

The title of this essay has become one of my favorite topics, both for discussion and writing, no doubt because of its elusiveness. For sure, my journey to a more peaceful life has been arduous at times. I wasn't raised in a peaceful household. On the contrary, it was fraught with intense tension, loud, daily arguments, many long silences, and constant uncertainties. Thus, I didn't embrace the idea of peaceful living until I had spent way too many years in the fast lane of dissension and fear-filled decisions. As a matter of fact, I didn't come to truly understand what it meant to experience peace until I added the study of *A Course in Miracles* to my daily 12-step recovery commitment.

My journey on the 12-step path began nearly forty years ago. The blessing of the course was added nearly thirty years ago. Sitting here today, writing about the trajectory of my life and all the successes I have had, seems almost unfathomable. How has this all happened? Why me? Or am I imagining it? At times like these I seem to be little more than an observer of my life. And yet I know I made each and every choice to do all that I did on the dangerous curves of my life, and fortunately, in the midst of chaos, I stopped long enough to undertake a new set of choices. It's been these choices that have made the joys and peaceful moments of my life possible.

But what do those peaceful moments look like? They are the moments I choose to say nothing rather than engage in an argument I was invited to. They are the moments I seek to see Spirit or "the Christ" (this is open for your interpretation) in the faces of people I am about to judge. They are the moments I sincerely ask for help to see a situation or a person in another way. They are the moments I know, without a shadow of a doubt, that my learning partners surround my every move, and they are present for the cultivation of my peace-filled benefit.

Lest you think that I live, day to day, in peaceful repose, let me assure you that my life is far from that. I am merely a practitioner of peace. Occasionally. More than occasionally, perhaps, but certainly not constantly. There are numerous times in every day that my ego holds sway over my behavior. No matter how many times I ask for help to see something differently or seek to reframe what I am preparing to say so that my words aren't harsh, I slip and slide full force into a trap set by my cunning, baffling, and powerful ego. At those times I simply choose to forgive myself and try again, knowing that every next moment is an opportunity to practice peace.

One of the glories of making a commitment to the practice of peaceful behavior is that it feels good. It feels honorable, respectful, and kind. And I'm convinced it adds benefit to the universe we share with seven billion other souls. I'm so grateful for the phenomenon of the butterfly effect. Adding positive or negative ions to the atmosphere each time we make a gesture to a person, react to a situation, or even simply think an unkind or harmful thought is a mighty idea. Making the commitment to be a purveyor of peaceful ripples is a worthy assignment indeed.

Over the last few years I have made more than a concerted effort to impart tools for peaceful living through the books I have written (www.womens-spirituality.com), and the workshops I have facilitated. And even though I share these ideas joyfully and sincerely, my own ego fails to adhere to that which I "preach" far too often. Embarrassingly often, in fact. And yet, I know, each day offers me another collection of moments in which to practice what I know to be true.

What follows is a handful of tools that will effectively change how you relate to the people and relationships in your life. I also know that nothing changes if nothing changes. Why not consider the importance of each tool in respect to one of your primary relationship partners, defining partners very loosely.

Envision the person you want or need to apply this tool to, and then imagine walking through an experience with them:

- Embrace powerlessness.
- Practice the thought, "I can choose peace instead of this."
- Choose carefully between the two voices in your mind. One is wrong. Don't honor it.
- Every person we encounter is a messenger. Honor him and the message.
- Sidestep chaos.
- Sidestep angry people. They are simply afraid. Love them.
- Seek reasons to be grateful.
- Ask: what can I bring to my relationships today?
- Forgiveness is our primary lesson.
- Nothing happens by accident.
- Surrender does not mean defeat. It means love.
- Repeat often: I am here only to be truly helpful . . .

This is just a smattering of the tools that are available to us if we want to experience more peace in our lives on a daily basis. I know that every time I try to control another person or the outcome of a situation, I have forgotten that I am here to be truly helpful. I know that loving those learning partners who seem hard to love is the very reason they have shown up in my life. I know that when I am feeling slow to forgive, it's because I want to deny that who I see is me.

A peaceful life is at our beck and call. The only question facing us is: how much do we want it? This is our final stage calling to us, I think. I want to go out singing. I want those who gather for my wake to say I brought them joy, that they always felt accepted in my presence, that they loved my sense of humor, but most of all that they appreciated my willingness to surrender a point rather than insist I was always right. Being a purveyor of peace is a noble undertaking.

If you were to go tomorrow, have you done all that you had hoped to do? If not, list those things in your journal and make a plan for completing each one.

And finally, what do you hope you "hear" others say at your wake?

67

Telling Your Secrets

Sometimes, the biggest secrets you can only tell a stranger.
—Michelle Hodkin

If my memory serves me well, I have never written an essay about secrets before. But I do believe that holding secrets can result in keeping us stuck in an unhealthy place. Do we need to tell everyone our secrets? Of course not. But finding someone we can confide in, a friend or even a stranger we may never see again, is the place to begin to lighten our burden.

What is it about secrets that cause such inner turmoil? There are probably as many reasons as there are secrets being protected, but my experience has shown me that a secret of any kind interferes with my peace of mind. Holding back information from others, unless it's information that would harm them, simply makes me feel dishonest, even when the information I'm not sharing isn't related to the people I'm with. Secrets can simply make the holder of them feel unclean. This may seem like a strange description of the residue of a secret, but it does have an impact, a heavy impact. At least on some of us. At least on me.

If you don't share this same reaction to secrets, count yourself lucky, for now, but someday you may be privy to a secret that disturbs you and you will better understand what I'm saying here. If that day comes, you can return to this essay and rediscover how to find the peace I discovered.

For the sake of this essay, let's assume you, like me, are left feeling ill at ease when harboring a secret. Besides telling someone about it, if that's too difficult to begin with, writing a note to the God of your understanding, sharing the secret in that way, will lighten the burden almost instantly. That's perfect, in fact, as a first step. And it might give you so much freedom that you never need to share the secret any further. If that's the case: hurrah!

Possibly this still seems like a strange topic for an essay in a book on living long, living passionately. On the contrary, it's my opinion that it's a perfect essay to ruminate over. Living peacefully into our later years is much more than just a worthy goal. From my perspective, it's as close to being mandatory as is possible. We deserve a peaceful final stage. In fact, we have deserved to live peacefully our entire lives. However, our egos got in our way too often . . . way too often. Actually, the ego is generally the culprit when we consider the birthplace of our secrets. And the ego fights to make us hostage to them. The good news is that we don't have to be hostage to anyone or anything unless we agree to be. Giving any secret the power to rule our lives is nonsense. Utter nonsense.

You might be wondering why I'm making an issue of secrets. After all, we have all had them. Most of us still have a few. However, when they prevent us from having open and honest exchanges with friends and strangers alike, we must address them. We must decide it's time to release them. Until we do, we are living in a very uncomfortable place. For those of us who want peace, it won't be attained if a secret is holding us hostage.

There is a path to freedom, however. It's one I have relied on successfully. Of course, my way won't be everyone's way, but if it appeals to you at all, go for it before you change your mind. Grab a piece of paper and a pen or maybe head to your computer. Then begin at the beginning. Tell the secret to whomever you envision, perhaps an imaginary person, or the God of your understanding, or perhaps the person you owe an explanation to. At this point, we haven't decided if we are going to send this message to anyone. At this point, we are simply getting relief from the power it's holding over us.

You may well discover, as I have, that just as soon as you begin telling the secret, it loosens its hold on you. Remember, there is only one thing you should not do, and that's harm anyone with the truth of the secret. What we are seeking here, what I am hoping you have been seeking throughout the essays in this book, are ideas for easier, more grace-filled living throughout the last few chapters of your life. We reached this stage as the result of lots of hard work, coupled with many successes and a few failures too. We deserve to be peaceful. We deserve freedom from conflict. We deserve to celebrate that we have lived well, helped others to live well too, and can now ever so quietly walk the path that has been laid out before us.

One of the things that can mar our journey is the secrets that still grip us tightly. Now is the time to get free. Now is the time.

Let me guide you with the following exercise:

First, quiet the mind for a few minutes. Ask the God of your understanding to come forth, bringing the secrets too. Listen as each one is lifted up to your heart. See it. Feel it. Seek the help you need to let it leave your mind. Know that when it's gone, it's gone forever. To bother you no more.

Send each one on its way, here and now.

Try to express, either in writing or pictorially, what freedom from secrets feels like to you. Feel free to share how this has been with others who may seem stuck. Passing on the tools to living in peace with our fellow travelers is a worthy gift. We all deserve it. And every time we give this gift away, we are benefitting the universe of seven billion souls. Hallelujah.

———————————

68

Living with Death

To the well-organized mind, death is but the next great adventure.

—J. K. Rowling

We went to the funeral today for a ninety-one-year-old man. He was the loving father of one of our dear friends. This Rowling quote fits his life and death to a T. As we all listened to the words of his children, it was easy to *see* not only the organized mind of the man, but also clear evidence of his strong faith and his absolute belief in life after death, an adventure he longed to experience with his wife who was already there. He had lived well, very purposefully, and always full of hope and admiration for his eight children and their mother Marge, before she passed.

Marge died eight years ago, and although Tom loved life, loved spending time with his three sons and five daughters and their families, particularly his many grandchildren, he was eager to rejoin Marge. In his final hours, he told his children she was in the room with them, and that he'd be leaving with her soon. She had been, and still was, the love of his life.

My husband and I felt honored to be on the periphery of this family, evidenced by our many invitations to be present on myriad special occasions. Over the years, again and again, we were privy to the important lessons each one of Tom's children had learned at the feet of both parents. Lessons about loving wholly, living purposefully, and being sincerely generous to those with less, as well as those with more. To give was the point of their lives, according to Tom. Joe said on our way home that he thought they were quite possibly the only truly functional family he had ever known. I couldn't agree more.

Since death will visit every one of us reading this book, just as it has visited many of our loved ones already, contemplating what it will look like actually brings me joy. Not every reader will share my perception, of course. Some of you may dread the inevitable. I know many who do. Others will simply fear the great unknown that surrounds death. However, finding a way to accommodate that which is heading toward us is something we have to do. And if not now, when?

There is no perfect way to get ready for death, of course. Each in our own way is the best way. What is true for each of us, though, is that we will meet death more easily if we move toward it with a willingness and a certainty that God will greet us in that moment of stepping into our *next great adventure*.

I spent most of my twenties and early thirties espousing the theory that God was dead. It was a popular notion among our friends, especially my first husband's graduate school colleagues. Believing in God was a weakness, they all thought. Even a sign of obvious stupidity. Bill had convinced me of that too. I so wanted to fit in with his friends that I adopted their ideas carte blanche and eagerly, lest I be judged as too naïve, *too uneducated*. I was *only* a third grade teacher, after all. I wasn't yet a PhD student. I never even asked myself, "Does this idea fit for me?" My struggle to be a valuable asset to his group was simply too great.

How thrilled I am to finally be comfortable as myself. Although it took me a long time to grow into the woman I am, I'm happy to say that arriving here was worth every single, sometimes scary, step I took. Surviving the hundreds of dark alleys and even darker bars has offered me a big payoff. I have shared about my alcoholism in other essays, so it doesn't need to be rehashed again. But I do want to stress that my alcoholism, drug addiction, and addiction to men, followed by my subsequent recovery, has been the path I needed to take to discover the presence of a Higher Power, the source who was always by my side, even when I emphatically denied his existence. Again and again.

What I have learned from my fellow travelers on the journey of recovery is that every single step I have taken from birth until now was carefully charted, and I participated completely in creating every encounter I've had on the path I've followed. Believing this gives me great joy and overwhelming relief. It also fills me with eager anticipation about the rest of my journey.

I believe wholeheartedly that each experience will be perfect, just as every experience already lived was perfect. I know I will safely enter my final chapter at the right time, with the right frame of mind, and the right friends will see me off. Better yet, the right friends will welcome me when I get there.

Having no fear about my final chapter is so freeing. In an interesting way, it even heightens my subtle longing for the final steps on my journey. Don't misunderstand—I'm not so eager I'd do anything to help the end come sooner. On the contrary, I believe it will come at the right time. Not before and not later than the perfect time. I believe the same is true for each one of you too.

Let me help you look at your expectations. And fears, if you have any. One thing I learned in Alcoholics Anonymous, and it's a fact I'm so grateful to have learned, is that we are never alone. We have never been alone. Even when we are unaware of God's presence, he is there and here, and everywhere we are. He will patiently wait in the wings, so to speak, until it's our turn to go. For certain, we will be called at the right time. Not one moment sooner. And for certain, he will lead the way home.

If this isn't your perspective, that's fine. (As we say in the rooms of recovery, take what fits and leave the rest.) However you see the end coming is perfect for you. Getting ourselves ready, in some manner, makes sense though. Don't you agree? Perhaps some exercises like the ones that follow will help you get ready, knowing full well that the end isn't likely imminent.

Being ready, being free of any encumbrances that may trouble you, particularly if there were situations between you and friends or family that left you feeling vulnerable and uneasy, is necessary, I think. The final journey will feel bumpy, for sure, if there are conversations that need to happen. That inner guide, call him or her whatever pleases you, always lets us know if we have work to do. Listen up!

———————————

Is there any unfinished business you need to take care of?

If yes, write it out or share it with an impartial loved one before addressing it with the person you had the experience with. Doing one or the other before talking to the learning partner will lessen any fear you might have. Getting free of your past is mandatory if you want smooth sailing forward. After all, this is the most important leg of the trip of a lifetime.

What kind of relationship have you most commonly experienced with the God of your understanding?

Are you interested in cultivating a deeper or a different kind of relationship?

If you answered in the affirmative, how do you envision it?

If James Lipton from The Actors Studio asked you what you hope to hear God say when you arrive at the pearly gates, what would it be?

What do you imagine you might say to him or her?

Has your anticipation about the final chapter changed at all since reading this essay and responding to these exercises?

After passing over, what do you hope to experience immediately?

Whom do you hope to see?

What would you say to your loved ones if you could convey a message from your new home to them?

What final thoughts are hovering around your mind right now?

What final things do you wish you had said to your loved ones? Fortunately, you have not passed over yet. Say what needs to be said now. Right now!

69

The First Day of Your Retired Life

It's been my experience to know many people who simply can't slow down. They can't move out of the fast lane. They seem drawn to the grindstone, fearing they will lose their value if they aren't producing. Do I dare to admit, here in a book that I'm writing, that I am struggling to escape this category, which is why I recognize it so well in others? I have certainly been told by many that a PhD and thirty books published add up to quite enough work. I don't have anything more to prove. I know that. Really, I do. But I can't imagine getting up someday and not heading to my study to work. Just one more workshop or one more book always seems to call my name. As a matter of fact, I have my next book noodling around in my head as I'm nearing the end of this book you are now holding in your hands. There is always something waiting in the wings. And actually, I love that about my life. I love my enthusiasm for continuing to share what cries out to be said.

I know many of you reading this understand full well what I'm talking about. You, too, feel conflicted about the next stage of your life. Are you ready to even consider slowing down? Hopefully, this doesn't offend you, but many of us were in jobs that were not very challenging or interesting. Or perhaps they were confusing, and thus way too stressful too much of the time. Our new occupation is to be attentive and kind to everyone we see throughout the day. Every single person! This is definitely a promotion for most of us. And it is a job we have the capability to perform.

Not everyone reading this has retired yet. Many are only contemplating what that will look like. But for all of you, I hope the exercises that follow will guide you when it is your time to step aside for the next generation to pick up the reins. You need not feel compelled to do them all, or any of them, for that matter. But I think they will help you see that your life will never be unimportant to the many who are on the receiving end of the gift you are offering.

Let's imagine that today is the first day of your retired life.

Upon arising, what do you envision doing? And what is the reason for doing that?

1. What do you expect to miss about the career you had?

2. Is there a way you can bring that part you miss into this new phase? If yes, explain. Create a scenario to help in the explanation.

70

The Serenity Prayer

God grant me the serenity to accept the things I cannot change, courage to change the things I can, and wisdom to know the difference.

—The Serenity Prayer, Reinhold Niebuhr

This prayer is near and dear to my heart. It's the first prayer I heard when I entered the 12-step rooms in 1974. I well remember that I didn't fully understand it at first. The idea of accepting things as unchangeable by me just didn't seem reasonable. I was certain I could change whatever *or whomever* I put my mind to changing. Alas, that has not been true. I have tried thousands of times to change others, probably tens of thousands of times. Fortunately, *though surprisingly to me,* I never succeeded. Not ever.

Had I succeeded in changing others, even one other, my work would never be done. There would be no space in my life for retirement if my job was to constantly be changing others. Or trying to, at least. Nor would I ever feel a moment's peace. The burdens would be many, just as many as there were people in my life. And they would be unending too, not counting the constant conflicts I'd be causing. Messing with the lives of others messes up everyone's life, but none more than one's own.

This prayer has given peace of mind to millions of people in 12-step rooms, not counting all the other millions elsewhere who quite sensibly learned to rely on it when the chaos in their lives was simply too great to be ignored. How interesting that a simple prayer can help us *spiritually ignore* that which is just too much for us. But indeed, that's how this prayer does its best work. Letting go of everything we can't control, which is, in fact, nearly everything in our lives, offers such relief; although at first it seems to make our lives even more difficult. Discovering the power of letting go is a huge gift. None greater, some would say. As would I.

Not only is this prayer about the attainment of serenity, it's about acknowledging wisdom, and our personal capability of recognizing it at the right time. What a powerful prayer. To break it down in a very few words, we are inspired to be courageous and to let go. Serenity becomes an immediate gift for doing so, and we get a glimmer of wisdom in the process. This awareness of wisdom stops us in our tracks. The prayer, said repeatedly, changes our life, and changes it immeasurably.

Because I don't know how many of you reading this book have a spiritual practice of some kind that gives you solace or guidance when you need it, I suggest we consider using the words of this prayer as sensible, simple suggestions for improving our lives. If for no other reason than to feel greater peace, use them. As I have already said, the tiny, though very subtle idea of letting go of people, places, and situations is a powerful notion to embrace. It offers us an instant awareness of relief. The giving up of the idea that we can (or should) try to change others, control them in any way, is folly. It has always been folly, and it is the very action that creates unwanted conflict between people. And nations too. Just watch the news for confirmation of this fact.

The second facet of the prayer, "Courage to change the things I can," requires taking responsibility for our actions, and our actions result from our thoughts. So the first assignment is to become willing to think through any action we might consider is a good one before making an attempt to implement it. This takes a maturity that really has very little to do with actual age.

It's a maturity that is honed by our willingness to go slow, resist impulsiveness, and then pause, yet again, before doing anything.

Courage to change what we can brings us face to face with how limited our abilities really are, day to day, in regard to the behavior of others. Being able to change only ourselves doesn't feel very fair. After all, we are confronted by so many people and myriad situations that need to be tweaked, even in a tiny way. How can it be that we have no power to change all that needs to change before our very eyes? Isn't its very presence the only indication we need that our work is just beginning?

The question that hounded me for years was, "Why shouldn't I exert my will on others?" I was sure I knew exactly what every person should do because my experiences had taught me so much. And for sure I knew how to manage any situation. I was *a born manager*, I thought. I had bosses who told me so. My profession proved it. The power I wielded was false, however. My title implied power, but it wouldn't have stuck if I had not been in charge of salaries and promotions too.

Fortunately, I was blessed with the guidance of others to see the rewards awaiting me when I limited my reins of management to myself, particularly in regard to my personal life. The realization also quickly rose to the surface of my mind that my attempt to manage anyone else caused unnecessary grief, to them and to me. Trying to change the unchangeable is exhausting. Unrewarding. And impossible. Giving up my attempts to change others freed me to live a richer, far more peaceful life. Everyone who lets go will reap these rewards too.

The third part of Niebuhr's prayer is perhaps the most rewarding of all. Wisdom. Wisdom to know the difference between what we can change and what we can't. Every aspect, even the tiniest of thoughts and actions, of our life is affected when we acquire *wisdom*, and it comes to all of us if we are willing to accept its terms. And its terms encompass the idea of

God; the willingness to experience serenity; the celebration of acceptance; the freedom of letting go; and the willingness to be courageous and aware. Implementing all these opportunities, *and I do mean opportunities,* as we pass through each day of living endows us with wisdom beyond measure; a knowing that is deep, rich, protective, and inspiring.

We need to celebrate our differences along with the ways in which our lives run parallel to each other. The point of this essay is to drive home the idea that help is available to every one of us if we seek it. We don't need to pray in a particular way. We don't need to pray to a particular God. In fact, we don't need to pray at all. All this prayer asks us to do is quietly let others be themselves and change, in ourselves, those beliefs and behaviors that would make our lives more peaceful. Pretty simple when you get down to the particulars. Isn't it?

———————

Now let's look at what might be changed in ourselves. If there is nothing that you want to change, bravo. Then use this time and space to write a short essay in your journal about the strengths and behaviors you possess that serve you well. For the rest of us, let's make a list of what we'd like to let go of in ourselves.

Perhaps to get you started, I'll give an example or two of changes I need to make in myself. What I need to let go of is my unneeded suggestions to my husband of how to drive (more like me, of course). I hate it when I do it, and yet I continue to do it.

Here is my promise to you: To the best of my ability, I will do this no more. I will practice WAIT. (This stands for Why Am I Talking?) In fact, this simple suggestion has applications far and wide in my life.

My next change is to relinquish my unkind judgments of others. Period. In AA we say, in regard to our judgments of others, "You spot it, you got it," which means that we see in others some aspect of ourselves. Not a very complimentary comment.

Now it's your turn. Let my examples serve to guide you.
I am . . .

But I want to be . . .

The prayer will help me in the following way.

I will return to this exercise one month from today and reevaluate myself.

Have I changed?

Do I like who I am now? Better than before? Why or why not?

What's next to change? And why?

The point of this essay and its accompanying exercise is to prove to ourselves that we are never too old to change. All we have to do is monitor our behavior, noticing very honestly our behavior, and then make a plan for changing how we would prefer interacting with the community around us. The old adage that you can't teach an old dog new tricks is absolutely untrue.

The final thought regarding the Serenity Prayer and the power it wields if we want to utilize it fully is this: nothing is beyond us when it comes to changing ourselves. And everything is beyond us if we are intent on changing others. We will never know serenity if we are mired in the fallacy that we can change others.

Go in peace and be grateful for the numerous opportunities to live contentedly in your own shoes, and with your eyes on the next step that is yours, alone, to make.

———————————

71

Your Life Philosophy

Whatever will be, will be. Que sera, sera.

—Lyrics made famous by Doris Day

Whatever will be is a philosophy, of sorts, that appeals to many. Actually, I think there are many levels of understanding inherent in these few words. To some it implies that free will, thus choice, plays no role at all in our lives. In other words, we have no responsibility for how our life is unfolding. To others, it's a willingness to simply surrender to whatever is in a very disengaged way, to go along with the crowd rather than making a thoughtful choice that might be a better choice for us.

I personally like the philosophy held by spiritual intuitive Caroline Myss. With such clarity, she outlines her belief system in her book *Sacred Contracts*. In that book, she says our lives perfectly reflect those encounters we "designed, i.e., quite explicitly contracted to have," while on the other side. Our life experiences here, then, are part and parcel of the choices we agreed to there before waking up here. In other words, each one of us arranged the orchestration of our lives, choosing who would be first chair in each section of the orchestra as our life unfolded. Each and every lesson, very much like an aria, arose on cue. Whatever is was very intentionally decided on by each party that was or is involved.

Adopting Myss's belief system gave me great peace from the very start. It has continued to give me peace every step of the way. No painful experience from my past had me long in its clutches because, from the moment I read *Sacred Contracts*, I accepted my part in each painful equation. Even when the experience was childhood sexual abuse, I more or less understood, with Myss's help, my own role in it, accepting it and the lesson that ultimately led to a profound awareness of forgiveness.

I'm not at all certain that I'd ever have known what real forgiveness was, except within the parameters of that abuse. What l learned has served me well. It has served very well many others too who came to me with similar painful experiences in their lives. Together we were all able to move forward. As a matter of fact, I personally believe that's the only reason we show up in each other's lives at all.

Because I don't know you (I only have a glimmer of what you might be like since you picked up this book), I can only assume you are interested in "revisioning" the future that is calling to you. Each one of us is being called, at this very moment, to make a mark on history, our own history and the histories of all those dear ones who surround us. The kind of mark we make is up to us, of course, but we must not assume that our role in life is irrelevant to anyone because of our age. It's quite relevant to everyone, in fact. We have always led relevant lives. Our imprint is everywhere we have ever been. Everywhere. Our impact has been felt universally. It's our job to acknowledge that, and to make sure we are imprinting that which we want to send forth, moment by moment.

What fun it is to grow old with at least a modicum of understanding of what our lives have been about. What fun it also is to knowingly move among the friends and family members we have decided to cultivate in this particular life. There have been no accidents. As I have said in many other essays, in many other books, in fact: we have never wandered accidentally anywhere. Our experiences were carefully charted by none other than ourselves.

When thinking about the song "Que Sera, Sera (Whatever Will Be, Will Be)," it's my belief that our lives were not as based on happenstance as the words of that song imply. We came here full of purpose. We are living very purposefully with each of the people we have met along the way. This will remain true until our purpose has been fulfilled. And not a minute before. What a kind and loving awareness that is. Even if you don't share my philosophy about how our lives are unfolding, the idea that our lives have meaning and purpose surely can't be distasteful. Accepting the idea that there is purpose to our lives simply makes getting up each day more palatable. If nothing more.

Because the real point of this essay, and every essay, is for you to evaluate and monitor who and where you are on your path through this life, the time has come for you to take stock once again. The easiest way to do this is to let me lead you through a series of questions. You know the answers. Absolutely. However, they may be somewhat buried because we don't always want to know who we really are, why we have done some of the things we have done, and what we may be contemplating about our future. Just remember, this evaluation is for you. And only you. If you want to share it with a loved one, that's your call.

———————

In a few words, how would you explain your life philosophy?

How did it develop?

In what positive ways has it served you?

Would you say most of your friends have the same or similar life philosophies?

As you turn this final corner of life, is there any reason to consider if this philosophy is the best one for you now?

Can you define for yourself and others what your primary purpose here has been?

Has it changed over the years? Explain in what ways if it has.

What do you think caused that change?

If you had the power to determine your purpose for the remainder of your life, what would it be?

Throughout your life, your encounters gave root to your lessons. What were those primary lessons, as you look back now? And even more importantly, who were the teachers?

In summary, who were you here to impact?

Who was here to effect change in you?

What do you recognize as your last bit of unfinished business?

If you could make one change in your life now, what would that be?

Why?

Do you feel prepared to "end" your journey now? Do you relish that idea, or are you afraid? Be honest. This is your journal. No one else needs to see it.

If there is still work to be done, what is it?

Who is the last person you hope to have an encounter with?

———————————

72

Recalling Your Life Lessons

Whether we are forty or seventy, or even fourteen, we pine over the fact that we don't know what our future holds. Will we be happy? Will we be rich? Will we find true love? Know peace? Have hope? Feel secure? Be healthy? Questions abound when we contemplate the unknown, and for every one of us, the future appears to be unknown.

There is another way to look toward the future, however. In fact, there are many other ways, but the one that appeals to me, and that has appealed to me for many decades now, is trusting that my future *is already known,* absolutely. It's already "in the bag;" *it simply hasn't been revealed to me yet.* It is unfolding right on time, however, link by link, in the perfect way. The way I laid it out before waking up here, in this body.

I am delighted that life unfolds in this way for everyone! So I believe. And you don't have to believe that it's true for it to be true. That's the best part. You can sit on the sidelines, so to speak, shaking your head in amazement, and your life will happen, will unfold before you, according to the plan. What an awesome realization.

Even though my perception of how life unfolds is anything but happenstance, getting ahead of myself does little more than create unneeded and unproductive anxiety. It's far better for me to trust that all is well. All will always be well. Leaving the future to the God of our understanding allows us to attend to the present completely. Actually, unless we are committed to the present, we are not in touch with the only moment that exists. The present moment is the only real moment there is, in fact. Life is simply a series of these moments. Period. Take notice. Now.

I know I have made the point about our deeply personal, very creative involvement in preplanning every experience we have while here in a number of earlier essays. That has been intentional. Even though it's an idea that some people resist, it's an idea that many eventually grow into, with time. I've had friends and workshop participants say, "How can it be that we design our experiences before being born?" My answer is simply, "If this perspective on how life unfolds satisfies Caroline Myss, a brilliant spiritual intuitive, it satisfies me." It's not my intent to twist anyone's arm, only to share what makes sense to me based on my experience, strength, and hope. I am convinced that the lessons I have learned were perfect for me and for the individuals I encountered both within each lesson and following each lesson. It's all been like clockwork. However, if you can't get your mind around Myss's philosophy, that's fine. Take what works for you and let the rest slide by.

Let's pause for a moment here so that you can revisit some of your lessons throughout your life. Some of the recent ones might be easiest to recall. Take a few, quiet moments and let them come to mind. When you feel ready, share in your journal what some of those lessons were, at least two or three of them. Can you guess why you needed these lessons? Can you see how they fit into other life experiences? Is there a thread leading from one to another?

It's my hope that revisiting our lives in this way can help us make choices about how we want our future to look. Was there one lesson, in particular, from any part of your past that seems, now, to be in a category all by itself? For instance, one lesson I received that proved to be profound almost beyond words was when I was meeting with one of my dissertation committee professors. Even though I referenced this in earlier essays, I think it bears repeating. Mr. G had had my dissertation for many weeks, but had not given me, or it, his approval. He avoided returning my calls when I tried to make an appointment with him. When he finally sat down with me, barely looking in my direction, he gruffly said I had to rewrite it. Every word of it!

How I managed to remain composed remains a mystery to me, even to this day. However, he did agree to go through the document with me to highlight his concerns. He posed questions that "I" honestly did not hear, and "I" gave answers that I likewise never heard. This exchange transpired for more than three hours, at which point he finally looked up and said, almost smiling, "I am satisfied. I will see you at the oral."

And now the lesson! Out of sheer terror I had fully surrendered to my Higher Power the task I was faced with, which was explaining my dissertation. And he handled it completely. I never again doubted that God could and would do for me whatever needed to be done. Staying out of the way was all that I needed to remember. That lesson has proven to be the most significant one I came here to learn. Unfortunately, I have had to be reminded of his abilities more than a few times.

We experimented with a timeline in an earlier essay. Let's do so again. Close your eyes, though not quite yet. Return to junior high or high school. Can you, following a few moments of quiet, recall the first significant lesson you experienced?

If so, write it in your journal (your memory need not be perfect).

What makes this a lesson, from your perspective?

Does it lead naturally into other lessons?

List a few of them.

It may not have seemed possible to discern the single thread that's running through your life, but there has been one. Perhaps you can see that now. Next, let's look closely at our relationships.

Have they been similar, one to another? Or were some significantly different? Explain in a few words.

How do you explain and evaluate the content of your most significant relationship(s)?

What's the lesson inherent in the content? Remember, you both agreed to it, on the other side. Of course you don't remember that encounter, but it occurred.

Just for fun, particularly if you think my perception regarding our preplanned encounters is malarkey, write, draw, or tell someone else what your expectations are for future encounters. Basing your guess on who has shown up in your past, and what you have done alone or with those people, write a story that reveals your life from this day forward. Keep this assignment fun. Also, be aware that we are the deciders of our fate.

Read this story to a friend for feedback. Study what you wrote for the purpose of discerning the lessons you scripted for yourself, here, in this short piece of writing.

My encounters.

My lessons.

My purpose now as my life is winding down.

Finally, I am most content with . . .

———————————

73

A New Challenge

The difference between what we do and what we are capable of doing would suffice to solve most of the world's problems.

—Mahatma Gandhi

At first read, Gandhi has seemingly provided a very simple solution to the ills of the world. His idea relies on each of us, all seven billion of us, regardless of age, giving a little bit more each day to making this a better world, a better world for every one of us. The flaw in that thinking is that some people are simply onlookers, not doers. Some are just more capable than others. Some people have the means to do more. Period. And the doers are stretched very thin because we have so many areas of the world that are experiencing dire problems. Fortunately, many onlookers are beginning to get the message that they must step up too. Becoming a doer carries with it bonafide esteem, a quality in short supply among the slackers, a quality that vastly improves their lives, in fact.

We each know the category we have snuggled into so comfortably in the past. And stepping outside our comfort zone isn't easy. But as the world's population grows, someone has to pick up the slack. The good news about that is that many of us who have closed the door on the all-demanding career are eager to sink our teeth into a new challenge. Are you one of these people? Is picking up the slack calling out to you?

How lucky we are that turning sixty-five doesn't require mandatory retirement. How lucky we are, in fact, that one can retire at a much younger age, or work into one's late eighties. No age defines us. No career defines us. We define ourselves. We always have. Where we go in this next, probably final, stage of life is anyone's choice. But since much is needed because the ills of the world are so great, any one of us who wants a second meaningful career can design one, now.

I'm sure you must realize that this second career, if that's what you are calling it, was very carefully scouted out before you were born into this lifetime. Nothing we have done here, or will ever do here, should completely surprise us. Perhaps our memory doesn't immediately recall the scenario we find ourselves in, but our cells knew where they were headed. Indeed, they will know when it's our time to move on. I hope you find this idea as exciting as I find it. I have in mind what I want to do next. Do you? And even though Gandhi put out the call for folks who wanted to solve problems, that's not a requirement for a long life. It's acceptable to play bridge or golf too. It's who we interact with in the years we spend here that matters. It's our behavior in those interactions that counts. We will be ushered in to the encounters we agreed to have. Worry not. What will be, will be. Remember: que sera, sera. All is always well.

If you are one of the fortunate many who wants to move on into a second (or maybe third or fourth) career, what do you imagine that might be? Though it was determined much earlier, *in that other place and time,* what do you, here and now, expect that assignment to be? The desire you had then remains unchanged. I think. The fun is in listening for the clues, being open to the signs, discerning where your plan is taking you before you get there.

Let's revisit our life and our many accomplishments here and now before taking on the challenge of our next, perhaps final, stage. When you look at your life in decades, what pops up first?

1 to 10 years old. (Don't pretend otherwise. You accomplished a few things in your childhood.)

10 to 20 years of age. (You made a few crucial discoveries in this decade.)

20 to 30 years. (Some of the accomplishments here might have involved others too.)

30 to 40 years. (Whatever your work was, you grew in significant ways.)

40 to 50 years. (What memory stands out the most in this decade? It's a good clue about what really inspires you. It will continue to inspire you.)

50 to now. (List every great idea you had in these last few years. List all the people you felt a special kinship with too.) The reason for this exercise is that it draws us into who we really were and are. Too often we overlook the finer points of who we became as the years passed. We too often observe others far closer than we observe ourselves.

I want you to shake off this exercise now. So let's pause, turn off our minds, let the past slide away for now. After resting for a few minutes, I want you to introduce yourself to an audience who knows nothing about you. Give an honest overview of who you were and how you seem now. Have fun.

What did you learn about yourself? Leave no stone unturned.

What was the easiest part of this last exercise?

What was the hardest?

Does anything here indicate what you might want to do in this next stage of fruitful living? I hope so.

Name it and describe it now. Are there people you need to contact to get your next show on the road? Make a plan now for the all-important implementation.

Congratulations on a job well done!

―――――――――――

74

What if You Had Six Months to Live?

If you were told you had six months to live, what changes would you immediately make in your life? What's stopping you from having the life you'd rather have right now?

We are nearly at the end of this book. By now, you have examined yourself pretty well. You have left few stones unturned, and you know that whatever your struggles in life have been, they were part of your specific agenda, and they were educational. Hopefully one of the most exciting aspects of your investigation has been your awareness now of what a good person you are. We have all made mistakes throughout our lives, but our goodness far outweighs our badness.

Every one of us has done the best we could with the information we had in whatever circumstance we found ourselves in. For that, we can and should be grateful. The same, of course, has been true of our parents, our friends, even our casual acquaintances— all those individuals we frequently sat in judgment of. Those times we unfairly judged them were only because we didn't understand the truth: that they were doing their best in that moment. Wisdom comes with willingness, open-mindedness, experience, and humility. Seldom is it available to the very young. Never will the totally absorbed understand it.

We have been influenced by, and have influenced, others in significant ways throughout our lives. That's why we met, of course. I've said this so many times already, but once more might be the tipping point for a few of you. So here goes. The following principles you can bank on always being true:

1. You met *all your counterparts* because you prearranged the meeting.
2. You needed the information your contact possessed to complete some phase of your journey.
3. Everyone has benefitted as the result of every encounter made by everyone, everywhere.
4. Whether we know one another or not, we benefitted all seven billion of us.
5. The butterfly effect wields its power even if we don't believe in the phenomenon.
6. There is a truth that goes far deeper than words can explain. The mind ascertains it, regardless.
7. There are no uncertainties in life. There are just minds who don't know everything yet.
8. There is a spiritual explanation for every circumstance.
9. We will fully understand this when our time to know it has come.
10. Our purpose, here, was decided before we arrived.
11. Our purpose will be fulfilled at the right time. We are moving toward that time every moment.
12. If it appears, at times, that we are switching horses midstream, it was planned that way.
13. If we are to continue with a new set of goals, in this final stage of life, we will feel the nudge.
14. Our trajectory has never gone off course. It never will.

Our lives have been meaningful, and they will remain so, regardless of how large or small we have chosen to live. All we need to do is listen, and our next direction will become apparent. But now let's get back to the topic of this essay. What would you need to let go of, or dispense with, if you only had six months to live? This isn't an easy topic, but that's primarily because we so commonly resist thinking about death, and we hate change. And yet making the final few months of life as rich and rewarding as we can is worth the effort we put into it. It really is an activity every one of us should consider pursuing, regardless of our health and expectations for a long life. Things can change *on a dime*, they say.

The son of a friend made a careless, though fateful, dive into a pond some years ago and has been a quadriplegic ever since. He is fulfilling his purpose, nonetheless. It simply is a purpose far different from the one he and his family had imagined. For all of us, the same has always been true. Whatever we are meant to do will find its way to us. We can't escape our assigned task. However, if we are involved in activities that don't feel beneficial now, and our closing moments are approaching, must we keep doing that which doesn't bring us peace, now? If we are not peaceful, the world around us isn't peaceful either.

Let's, together, make some decisions about what we need to let go of. Doing it in tandem with others, even though we are not sharing the same space, is more comforting. I'll pose some key questions. You think on them a while, and then honestly answer them to the best of your ability. There are no wrong answers. Nor are there any absolutely right ones. Every answer is contingent solely upon your circumstances. And you can change your mind.

Here goes:

What do you dread doing? Write that down and commit to no longer doing it. Maybe it's having dinner with certain people you feel obliged to entertain. You can stop now. Or maybe it's paying the bills. Turn them over to your spouse.

What have you always said you'd like to do someday?

Play an instrument? Do a five hundred–piece puzzle? Write letters to individuals you greatly admire? Do it. Before your time has run out.

Where had you always hoped to go before you died? Google it now. And if your spouse doesn't want to go, go anyway. Take a friend.

What is the unfinished business in your life? Do you need to make amends? Begin making the calls or writing those letters. Now.

Now think about those who you love and will be leaving. What haven't you said that you want to say? Now is the time.

It's certainly my hope that you haven't experienced this exercise as maudlin. Looking at the end of our time wearing these skins can be viewed as preparation for the inevitable. Tying up loose ends can be freeing, hope filled, and spiritually satisfying. Being prepared for whatever the final days may be quiets the soul. I think. At least I'm contented by this process. I intend to exercise this process when my notice comes.

And now one last exercise. What have been the best parts of your life?

Notice I said "parts." I want you to think, to meditate for more than a few moments with this question rolling around in your mind. Then come back to this page, and your journal page, and put your thoughts in black and white. Don't let them get away. They are deserving of your attention, your last moments of appreciation. Your thanks, so to speak.

And now we head to our final essay. Number 75.

75

Enthusiasm

We act as though comfort and luxury were the chief requirements in life, when all we need to make us really happy is something to be enthusiastic about.

—Charles Kingsley

I chose this quote for the final essay in the book because it rang so quietly true. I actually didn't know who Charles Kingsley was, so I did what so many of us do, and I googled him. I learned that he lived in the mid-1800s and that he was a novelist and a Christian Socialist. What I read about him as a man and great thinker of his time appealed to me, and the above quote, in particular, called out.

I think enthusiasm for some element in our life is the key to having the desire to get up every day. And as the years pass, particularly as we enter what, for me, has become the final stage of life, I know I must have passion for doing something not attempted before, or I must work to enhance a skill already present to keep my enthusiasm churning. I can't simply do over and over again what I have already done so many times before. This doesn't mean that what I have spent my life doing has lost its value. On the contrary. It only means that at some point, enthusiasm wanes. I have seen it happen to others. And I know I am no different. Making a decision to explore new territory is the impetus I think most folks need to get up daily with enthusiasm when we age.

My husband's passion is to know more about virtually any topic he hears just a smidgen about. He is the most curious person I have ever met. His curiosity, in fact, is what attracted me to him some forty years ago. He also has a remarkable capacity for remembering all that he has read or watched. He simply never tires of wanting to know more. His enthusiasm for the ordinary makes it seem extraordinary when he retells their story. And people are eager for his stories. I have observed this throughout our marriage. Our eagerness to know more feeds his desire, I think.

Because some of you are on the precipice of entering this final stage right along with me, the choices you may need to make about many elements of your life are only now passing through your mind. Some of these choices relate to changes in housing. Some will relate to changing locations, even. I actually know hundreds of couples and singles who have moved to a new part of the country for the final stage of life. For some that move was financial. For others, it had to do with health or weather or the movement of children or friends. And for a few, it was the basic drive for a new adventure. The good news is that we can always move back home again. No decision has to be made forever.

Getting older doesn't necessarily mean leading a quieter life. However, it may be slower in certain respects. I know, at seventy-five, that I don't have the energy I had at sixty. I observed this firsthand just a week ago when my niece, who is sixty, was visiting with her husband. Taking a morning walk together made it obvious that I no longer power-walked at her speed. The rest of the week she walked before I got up. I had to laugh. This was me a few years ago when I walked with my older sisters.

She and I went shopping and I experienced another example of the age difference. She bought me an e-cloth, a new method for washing windows, as a hostess gift. When we got home, I was ready to rest a while. She, on the other hand, excitedly washed every window in my house, both inside and out, screens too, without even breathing hard. Almost without stopping to eat. I was nearly exhausted just watching her. Her joy at offering this as an additional gift to me was all the sustenance she needed.

Did I do that at sixty? It's doubtful. I never liked housework, but I do know I burned the candle at both ends very success-fully for many years, a feat that's thankfully behind me now. That section of my chart has been completed.

The present fills me with the same kind of healthy anticipa-tion I have felt ever since I entered a 12-step room forty years ago. Being able to trust that life was going to be full of oppor-tunities I would be grateful for was such a gift, an unexpected gift. That's not the expectation I had lived with during the first thirty-six years of life. Then I was always waiting for the other, heavier shoe to drop. And on my head! I had not yet acquired the wisdom that my life had been charted already, and by me, no less. What a mind-blowing and spiritually satisfying con-cept this was to acquire. It pleases me every time I pay it some attention.

And here I sit, writing the last essay of this book. Know-ing that I planned this too, before coming into this experience, gives me such a sense of awe. You may not cotton on to this belief system, but it's very satisfying to me. At an earlier stage of my life I lived in fear. I lived in constant fear about the future, about abandonment, about whatever experience I was having at the time. Now I fully trust that whatever is happening is by my choice. Whoever I am having the experience with chose it also. Perhaps you will never find this belief system of interest or comfort to you. And that's okay. But if I could, I'd try to con-vince you to try it on for just a week so that you can see how it can change your experiences and your perception of the people and circumstances in your life.

Just because we are closing in on a later stage of life, per-haps even the final stage as I imagine I am entering, wandering into it with healthy anticipation and ripe enthusiasm will absolutely make the experiences sizzle with meaning. Seem naïve? Perhaps. Personally, I think not. It's comforting and assuring to me. Nothing I wander into is unprepared for me. This idea eases every step I take. Wherever I go, I have been expected by everyone who is or was waiting there for me. This truth makes me want to jump for joy.

When I look over my life, I gladly now know these experiences and specific individuals, among a host of others, were chosen to be present on my timeline. Without them, I'd not be here, doing what I do. I'd like to review them for my benefit. Perhaps for yours too. They are my assurance that the remaining years will be just as rich and specifically planned for:

1. My longing for connection as a child.
2. My experience of sexual abuse before my teens.
3. My first drink at thirteen.
4. My acting out in high school.
5. My first serious boyfriend at fifteen.
6. My college and sorority years.
7. My marriage to Bill.
8. The infidelities.
9. My years teaching at an inner city school.
10. The divorce.
11. The wild years while in grad school.
12. Getting into recovery.
13. Meeting Joe.
14. Completing my PhD.
15. Working at Hazelden.
16. Writing my first book.

17. The hundreds of workshops.
18. The list of published books continuing to grow.
19. The lessening energy.
20. The continuing enthusiasm.
21. The desire for new goals has been seeded.
22. The fertilization process is at hand.

Even though you may not share what I will call, "the Caroline Myss explanation of how our lives unfold," make a list like mine naming those events and people who ushered you to where you find yourself now.

What has your trip included?

We will awaken tomorrow and every day after that with eagerness to continue the journey if that's what we have set our minds to do. My belief system has prepared me to continue the journey that reflects the choices I so thoughtfully made long ago, before memory began. I may not like each of them initially, but as soon as I am willing to remember that I did ask for this one too, all will be well. Grabbing hold of the spiritual philosophy that says we are where we have asked to be, that there are no accidents, and that the people we need will show up here too is a mighty leap of faith for the uninitiated. I am so grateful that I was willing to make it. And as I have repeatedly said throughout this book, to any who are nonbelievers, once you step out into the unknown, it will meet you and lift you to safety. Hallelujah.

May you go forth in peace, knowing you go where you are needed. The one assignment we all share, no matter our age, our gender, our spiritual affinity, is to add a moment's worth of peace to every person we encounter. With each encounter, the entire universe moves closer to the tipping point where peace is all there is. Doing our part each day gives all the meaning we ever really need to living each day to its fullest. Enthusiasm will be reborn in us with every kindness we pass on to the next eager soul.

God bless you, one and all.

About the Author

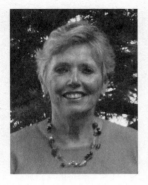

Karen Casey is a writer and workshop facilitator. She works with 12-step recovery workshops, with women in all stages of their life journeys, and, most recently, with people who are navigating their later stages of life. Her first book *Each Day a New Beginning: Daily Meditations for Women,* a classic for women in recovery, was first published in 1982. It has sold more than 3 million copies. She has published more than two dozen books since then, among them *Change Your Mind and Your Life Will Follow; The Good Stuff from Growing Up in a Dysfunctional Family; Codependence and the Power of Detachment; Let Go Now: Embracing Detachment;* and *Peace a Day at a Time.*

Living Long, Living Passionately: 75 Ways (and Counting) to Bring Peace and Purpose to Your Life is a very personal book, something of a birthday gift to herself and to her friends and followers. In it she explores the many ways we can live in the present, learning from and celebrating the past, giving up regrets, and experiencing peace, passion, and purpose each and every day.

Karen and her husband Joe divide their time between Naples, Florida, and Prior Lake, Minnesota, in addition to spending time near Lafayette, Indiana, her hometown. Casey travels throughout the United States and internationally, carrying her message of hope and peace. She is a sought-after speaker at such venues as the international A Course in Miracles conference. Visit Karen online at *www.womens-spirituality.com.*

To Our Readers

Conari Press, an imprint of Red Wheel/Weiser, publishes books on topics ranging from spirituality, personal growth, and relationships to women's issues, parenting, and social issues. Our mission is to publish quality books that will make a difference in people's lives—how we feel about ourselves and how we relate to one another. We value integrity, compassion, and receptivity, both in the books we publish and in the way we do business.

Our readers are our most important resource, and we appreciate your input, suggestions, and ideas about what you would like to see published.

Visit our website at *www.redwheelweiser.com* to learn about our upcoming books and free downloads, and be sure to go to *www.redwheelweiser.com/newsletter* to sign up for newsletters and exclusive offers.

You can also contact us at *info@rwwbooks.com*.

Conari Press

an imprint of Red Wheel/Weiser, LLC
665 Third Street, Suite 400
San Francisco, CA 94107